Callous Disregard

Autism and Vaccines—The Truth
Behind a Tragedy

Andrew J. Wakefield

Skyhorse Publishing

NOTE TO ALL CUSTOMERS:

NOT FOR SALE IN THE UNITED KINGDOM

10 9 8 7 6 5 4 3 2 1

Paperback ISBN: 978-1-61608-323-6

Library of Congress Cataloging-in-Publication Data

Wakefield, Andrew J.
Callous disregard: Autism and vaccines—the truth behind a tragedy /
Andrew J. Wakefield.
p. ; cm.
Other title: Autism and vaccines—the truth behind a tragedy
Includes bibliographical references.
ISBN 978-1-61608-169-0 (hardcover : alk. paper)
1. Autism in children--Etiology. 2. MMR vaccine--Side effects. I. Lancet. II.
Title. III. Title: Autism and vaccines—the truth behind a tragedy.
   [DNLM: 1. Autistic Disorder--etiology--Personal Narratives. 2. Child. 3.
Health Policy--Personal Narratives. 4. Measles-Mumps-Rubella Vaccine--adverse
effects--Personal Narratives. WM 203.5 W147c 2010]
   RJ506.A9W353 2010
   618.92'85882071--dc22
                        2010017228

Printed in Canada

This book is dedicated to
my inspirational and long-suffering wife,
Carmel, and to our wonderful children,
James, Sam, Imogen, and Corin
– cherish your minds and use them well.

Acknowledgements

I would like to express my enormous gratitude to those directly involved in the production of this book. They include my wife, Carmel; my editor Teri Arranga; my designer Fiona Mayne; Jim Moody with whom I co-wrote "Ethics, Evidence, and the Death of Medicine," which appears as the afterword to this book; Dr. Carol Stott who assisted with Chapter 1; Polly Tommey for her support and allowing access to her team and permission to reprint articles from *The Autism File*; the editors of *Age of Autism* for permission to reprint Chapter 13; Wendy Fournier for designing the website www.callous-disregard.com; and all of those individuals and organizations that have provided a link to this website. I am particularly grateful to Dr. Peter Fletcher, Jenny McCarthy, and Jim Moody for their commentaries as well as those providing additional remarks. My thanks are also due to Tony Lyons of Skyhorse Publishing and to Kim Stagliano for making the introduction.

Beyond this is an army of supporters and fellow travelers to whom I am related by blood, sweat, and tears; my sincere thanks are extended to you also.

CONTENTS

i   Preface

iii   Foreword

v   Dramatis Personae

1   Why

3   Prologue: Callous Disregard

9   That Paper

25   The Children

49   The Dean's Dilemma

65   The Whistleblower

77   Ethics and the Masses

83   The Dean's Press Briefing

101   Horton and *The Lancet*

117   Horton's Evidence

133   The Devil's in the Detail

143   Bedlam or Bonaparte

169   Disclosure

181   Deer

223   Poisoning Young Minds

233   Afterword: Ethics, Evidence and the Death of Medicine

247   Epilogue

250   Timeline

267   Postscript

271   Biography

PREFACE

Letter from Dr. Peter Fletcher, Ex-Principal Medical Officer with responsibility for the UK's Committee on Safety of Medicines and later Senior Principal Medical Officer and Chief Scientific Officer

My first comment on this excellent book is in respect of whether or not this whole catastrophe could have been avoided by action taken years earlier than *The Lancet* paper. By about 1987 in the UK, product licence (PL) submissions for three MMR vaccines had been initiated and were the subject of discussion by the Joint Committee on Vaccination and Immunisation (JCVI). My past position of Principal Medical Officer with responsibility for the main Committee on Safety of Medicines (CSM) and its sub-Committees leads me to the conclusion that a great deal could have been done.

It would have come to my attention from minutes of the JCVI that they were urging rapid granting of PLs for the three vaccines. That news would have been alarming because the JCVI was a purely advisory committee (i.e., not a Section 4 committee under the Medicines Act) and had no powers in the granting or refusal of PLs.

In the past there would have been no way in which the CSM would have recommended the granting of PLs on such scanty evidence of safety in the submissions. By 1988/9 the only evidence available was a handful of clinical trials each having no more than 7-800 subjects and none of them conducted in the UK. Had I still been there I would have required at least 10,000 patients in each submission with active safety surveillance for a minimum of 3 months with the possibility that this could be extended if untoward findings should be reported.

This would most probably have solved our current problem as we now know that at least 35 cases of "autism" had been officially reported by about 1993.

My second comment is to emphasise the great importance of the "positive rechallenge" cases which, for all practical purposes, prove causality. The CSM has always accepted that positive rechallenge in the absence of other equivalent and credible causes has to be accepted as a causal relationship.

i

My third comment concerns the analysis of anaphylaxis as a serious adverse effect. This has been much neglected and carefully avoided when mortality of vaccines is discussed. This is of primary importance when benefits and risks of vaccination are considered and compared with mortality of infections. If, for example, pre-vaccination figures for annual mortality due to measles (about 50 in 1967) are to be compared with annual mortality due to vaccines then, in developed countries where improvements in social conditions and standards of health care have been achieved, the differences become uncomfortably close.

My fourth comment relates to the safety evaluation of medicinal products intended for healthy people. The two biggest examples are hormonal contraceptives and vaccines. The differences between the two are mind-boggling. The contraceptives have been evaluated more intensively than any other group of medicinal products both in humans and animals. In contrast, vaccines have been minimally investigated and there seems to be no hope of an improvement in the future.

My fifth comment is related to the overall conduct of the GMC* case. I have now been involved in five different legal cases, and in all I have been in varying levels of despair when faced with the medical and scientific ignorance of the lawyers (solicitors and barristers) on both sides. This is quite understandable since a medical education extends over many years and, although the lawyers do quite well on the specifics of the case, they are lost when it comes to the bigger picture. This is referred to very nicely on page 143 with Charcot et al., and to some extent, it excuses the overall feeling of the case descending into an undignified catalogue of bickering between very irritating academics.

Lastly, I would like to mention the general clinical picture(s) presented by these children which, in my view, constitutes a complex new syndrome. The differing clinical observations cannot each have a different and separated pathological cause. It may be that two or just possibly three different pathological processes are involved, but the root cause has to be a single initiating factor – almost certainly vaccines.

* *General Medical Council vs. Wakefield, Walker-Smith, and Murch*

FOREWORD

I'm so glad Andy Wakefield finally has the chance to tell his story. Perhaps no debate on the planet right now is more confusing, more conflicting, or more maddening for parents than the debate over the causes and treatments of autism.

As the parent of a child who regressed into autism after his vaccinations, I have always considered Andy Wakefield to represent the kind of doctor and scientist who will ultimately help us end the epidemic of children with autism.

If you understand Andy's story completely, I think you will quickly realize that he did the sort of thing most of us expect out of our doctors and something most of us were taught by the time we were in kindergarten: he listened closely to the stories of parents and he told the truth.

I really wish the primary trigger for autism was something everyone could dislike like cigarettes or rat poison. It would make ending this epidemic so much easier. Unfortunately, it appears that a product intended for good—vaccines—also has a dark side, which is the ability to do harm in certain children. This ability to do harm has unfortunately increased quite a bit in the last few decades because children today receive so many more shots than when most parents were kids.

I understand that a portion of the population will continue to believe that all of us parents are crazy and that vaccines couldn't possibly do any harm. I really wish some of these people could have sat with me through the thousands of conversations I have had with parents of children with autism who have all told me the same story: their child was developing normally, and after each vaccine appointment things got worse until they ended up with autism. You hear this story once, it's disturbing, a dozen times it starts to feel like a pattern, a thousand times and you begin to wonder why this is still a debate.

Andy Wakefield did the same thing. He listened to parents who reported two things: their children with autism were suffering from severe bowel pain, and the children regressed into autism after vaccination. He listened, he studied, and he published what he learned.

I believe history will be very kind to Andy Wakefield. For the moment, he is the symbol of a very unfortunate reality, a reality that a medical system trying to do good may have done just the opposite. With time, I believe he will also be the symbol of someone who stood up for truth, despite extreme pressure to stand down.

For hundreds of thousands of parents around the world, myself included, Andy Wakefield is a symbol of strength and conviction that all parents of children with autism can use to fight for truth and the best lives possible for their kids.

Jenny McCarthy
April 22, 2010
Los Angeles, CA

DRAMATIS PERSONAE

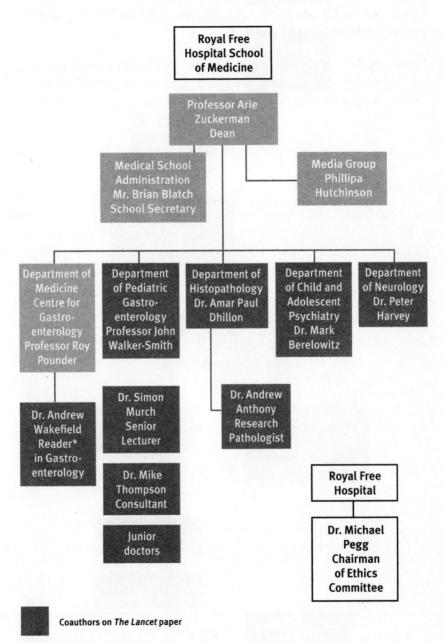

Royal Free Hospital School of Medicine

Professor Arie Zuckerman
Dean

Medical School Administration
Mr. Brian Blatch
School Secretary

Media Group
Phillipa Hutchinson

Department of Medicine Centre for Gastroenterology
Professor Roy Pounder

Department of Pediatric Gastroenterology
Professor John Walker-Smith

Department of Histopathology
Dr. Amar Paul Dhillon

Department of Child and Adolescent Psychiatry
Dr. Mark Berelowitz

Department of Neurology
Dr. Peter Harvey

Dr. Andrew Wakefield
Reader* in Gastroenterology

Dr. Simon Murch
Senior Lecturer

Dr. Andrew Anthony
Research Pathologist

Dr. Mike Thompson
Consultant

Junior doctors

Royal Free Hospital

**Dr. Michael Pegg
Chairman of Ethics Committee**

Coauthors on *The Lancet* paper

* Roughly equivalent to associate professor in US.

v

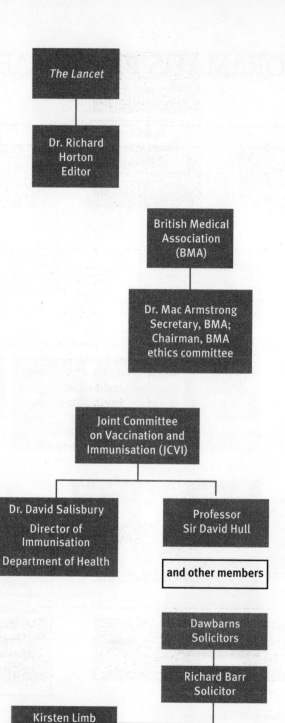

The Lancet

Dr. Richard Horton
Editor

British Medical Association (BMA)

Dr. Mac Armstrong
Secretary, BMA;
Chairman, BMA
ethics committee

Joint Committee on Vaccination and Immunisation (JCVI)

Dr. David Salisbury
Director of Immunisation
Department of Health

Professor Sir David Hull

and other members

Dawbarns Solicitors

Richard Barr
Solicitor

Kirsten Limb
Paralegal

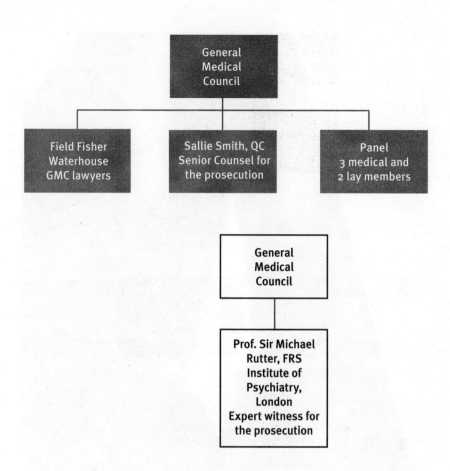

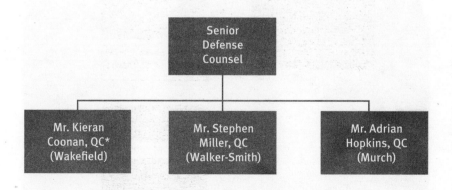

* Queen's Counsel

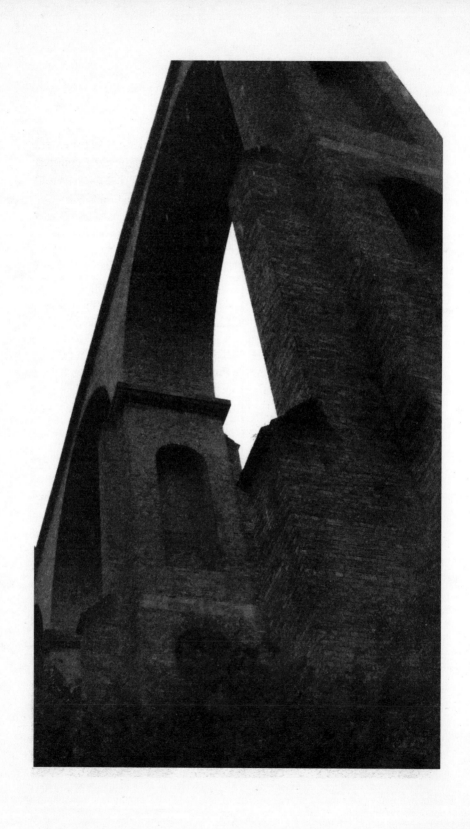

Why

Another north-easterly wind insinuated its futile energies between the massive brick piers of Hounds Ghyll viaduct. Although the wind endured, the earlier downpour had turned to a light drizzle – light for County Durham, in the far north of England – as their journey came to an end.

As if for the first time, Mark seemed attuned to his mother's sense of purpose and he offered no resistance. He did not scream, or fight, or hit himself in the face; he did not bite his scarred and scabby arms or suddenly collapse to the ground as if invisible guy-ropes could no longer hold him. Instead, entranced by the raindrops and in awe of the viaduct's ordered brickwork, he mouthed in silent wonder at it all. At the mid-point of the viaduct she turned to the north, the deep valley before her – in places its walls sheer, glistening black, cut by relentless waters that were now barely visible in the fading light far, far below. Mark looked up into his mother's face; beyond its years, alone, harassed, pursued, and he understood her unhappiness. He loved her, although he had no way – no wiring – that allowed him to express this.

With the aid of some old timbers she helped him onto the parapet, her grip so firm that it hurt them both. This was the hardest part, the lichened stone wet and perilous, her fear of heights. Standing there at last, against the wind and against the world, he looked at her and she at him. "No," she thought, "this is the hardest part." Without a word, without another thought she stepped into oblivion, her most precious possession taken with her, to rank in death with Egyptian queens. They were not equal to the wind and in one final effort it gusted into them, threatening to smash the waif-like Mark into the merciless viaduct. She knew. She was ready. Falling ever faster, she pulled him to her, love and instinct keeping him safe.

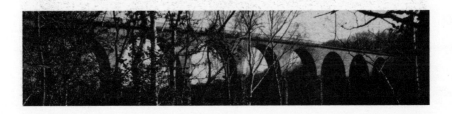

PROLOGUE

Callous Disregard[1]

If autism does not affect your family now, it will. If something does not change – and change soon – this is almost a mathematical certainty. This book affects you also. It is not a parochial look at a trivial medical spat in the UK, but dispatches from the battlefront in a major confrontation – a struggle against compromise in medicine, corruption of science, and a real and present threat to children in the interests of policy and profit. It is a story of how "the system" deals with dissent among its doctors and scientists.

This book is composed of a series of essays that deal with the now infamous paper – a humble case series – written by doctors at the Royal Free Hospital and published in *The Lancet* in February 1998.[2] The essays were originally intended to stand alone and some repetition is inevitable.

The Lancet paper described the clinical history and findings in a group of 12 children, referred to in these essays as *The Lancet 12*. The children presented with autistic regression and gastrointestinal symptoms. When investigated diligently and appropriately, they turned out to have intestinal inflammation, and there are reasons to believe that this inflammation may, in turn, be linked to their neurological disorder. Thus, the paper captured the essential elements of a new disease syndrome – a potentially treatable syndrome – and that should have been cause for some small celebration. Had the children's regression followed natural chicken pox, this book would never have been written. It didn't; for nine children (as it turns out), behavioral changes and subsequent developmental regression followed exposure to the MMR vaccine and thereby hangs this tale.

In the spring of 1982, I was a very junior doctor, undertaking my second 6-month rotation as a houseman (intern) in medicine at St. Mary's Hospital, my alma mater, in Paddington, West London. Taking a brief walk outside at lunchtime to get a sandwich, I heard a huge explosion. Immediately, instinctively, I knew it was a bomb.

At that time, hostilities in Northern Ireland had intensified, and disaffection within the ranks of the Irish Republican Army had led to the formation of the more militant Irish National Liberation Army. All at once there was movement; I found myself bundled into the back of an ambulance and headed at breakneck speed to who-knows-where. The ambulance man in the passenger seat shouted back to the two nurses and me that we were headed for a bombing in Regent's Park. In a muted effort at professionalism, we went through an inventory of the equipment we had available; in truth, we were terrified.

The scene in Regent's Park had a surreal quality. Against the backdrop of a gentle English summer's day, the bandstand and the band of the regiment of Royal Green Jackets had been blown to pieces. Sheet music blew among flattened deck chairs and fallen bandsmen. The bomb had been placed under the floorboards in the center of the bandstand. Such were the kinetics of the explosion that those sitting on top of the bomb had been blown up to 50 feet away, while mercifully, those not 3 yards away "escaped" with perforated eardrums and shock.

As it turned out, all but a few of the injured had already been evacuated and only a few soldiers with minor injuries remained, awaiting transport to hospital for a check-up and eardrops. There was nothing for us to do, save tour the devastation with a senior member of the emergency services to declare as dead blackened limbs and torsos.

When it came time to leave, I turned one last time before climbing back into the ambulance. I did so in order to reinforce that I should never forget what had happened that day. I felt an overwhelming sense of futility and failure; my medical training had counted for nothing, there was nothing to be done — nothing. In contrast, when in 1995 I was approached by Rosemary Kessick, portending the first ripples of the coming autism tsunami, I determined that there just might be something I could do. And so I did because something is more than nothing.

What has happened in the meantime is a story that was written long before any of us were born. It is the story of how the powerful deal with threats to their interests. It was recently suggested to me in an interview with a major US network that this was really just conspiracy theory. As it happened, earlier that week, internal memos from the pharmaceutical giant Merck were disclosed to the Australian court in the Vioxx litigation. They talked of how Merck had to "neutralise" dissent from those doctors who questioned the safety of this drug. In relation to these concerned doctors, one of the e-mails read:

We may need to seek them out and destroy them where they live.[3]

It would seem that rather than being conspiracy theory, this can sometimes be corporate policy.

To the vaccine industry, the regulators, public health officials and doctors, pediatricians, and Bill and Melinda Gates,[7] I would say this: the success of vaccination programs requires the willing participation of consumers. Key to any success, therefore, is public confidence in the scientists, doctors, and policy makers (including industry) that shape these programs. In turn, the key to that confidence is a safety first vaccine agenda. Those whose priority is *safety first* are not anti-vaccine. By analogy, those who ordered the recall of multiple Toyota brands for sticking gas pedals are not anti-car. The following from the *Examiner* may provide some context:

> ### Toyota Recall
> *An investigation by the Federal government has uncovered what appears to be presentation documents from July of 2009 where Toyota boasts about saving $100 million because they were able to negotiate a limited equipment recall for the Toyota Camry and Lexus ES vehicles instead of a more serious and costly problem with the cars. The point was listed under a section called "wins."*

The federal regulators, the National Highway Traffic Safety Administration (NHTSA), had this to say about Toyota:

> *Safety is everybody's responsibility... It's not just the federal government's job to catch safety defects... It's the responsibility of automakers to come forward when there is a problem. Unfortunately, this document is very telling... we're going to hold Toyota's feet to the fire and make sure they do what's necessary to make their cars safe for the driving public.*[4]

Who, here, is ultimately anti-car or, to be more specific, anti-Toyota brand car? In a free market, without mandates, what has happened at Toyota is unlikely to boost public confidence and, therefore, the company's sales and profitability. Liability for deaths and injuries is likely to haunt them for many years to come.

And what about the complicity of ex-regulators?

> ### Toyota Used Ex-Regulators to Help Kill Probes[5]
> *Toyota (TM) hired ex-government regulators to kill at least four investigations into problems with its cars in the U.S.*

Those who are a threat to public confidence, those who do not mandate a *safety first* agenda, are the greatest threat to the vaccine program; *they* are ultimately anti-vaccine.

So, where do *you* – the regulators and the vaccine industry – stand in 2010 with *your* costly PR programs; *your* ruthless, pragmatic exorcism of dissent; *your* public confidence rating?

Study: 1 in 4 parents think vaccines cause autism[6]
A new study says that 54 percent of parents are worried about serious adverse effects caused by vaccines, and 25 percent of parents believe that vaccines can cause autism.

You have failed.

To the parents I would say, trust your instincts above all else. When considering how to vaccinate your children, read, get educated, and demand fully informed consent and answers to your questions. When you are stonewalled or these answers are not to your satisfaction, trust your instinct. I say this as someone who has studied and engaged in the science and who has become aware of the limitations of our knowledge and understanding of vaccine safety issues. Maternal instinct, in contrast, has been a steady hand upon the tiller of evolution; we would not be here without it.

As corroboration of this instinct, it may not come as a surprise that as a matter of fact, the US vaccine court began compensating for cases of vaccine-caused autism starting in 1991,[8] and the US Department of Health and Human Services has been secretly settling cases of vaccine-caused autism without a hearing also since 1991. For example, we offer the following from cbsnews.com:

> As CBS News has reported, the government has been settling vaccine injuries that resulted in autism and/or autistic symptoms since at least the early 1990's, while at the same time telling the public there is no cause for concern. Not all of the cases are published, but some of them are and can be found by searching legal case databases.[9]

Nontheless, questioning the safety of a vaccine led, by twists and turns, to a disciplinary hearing for me and two coauthors of The Lancet paper before the UK's medical regulator, the General Medical Council (GMC). During the GMC hearing, I went back to Regent's Park — to the crime scene. It was winter; there was no band, no music, and no children running among deck chairs. There were no deck chairs. But for all that, you could not have guessed at the history of this place. And as I was leaving, I turned, and there were bodies everywhere. I looked back, not in anger, but with almost the same sense of futility and failure that I had felt some time before. We cannot allow ourselves such feelings; there is a job to do.

What follows was written in the teeth of the storm. It might have been the log of a doomed captain written in the cabin of a war-torn frigate, tacking on shredded sails, running from another – perhaps final – broadside. But it is not; it was written from the bridge, the helm secure, the wind at our backs, and the sails full as the aggressor slips back below an uncertain horizon. The day will belong to Reason.

Endnotes

[1] At the GMC I was accused and found guilty of "callous disregard" for the suffering of children.

[2] Wakefield, AJ, Murch SH, Anthony A, Linnell J, Casson DM, Malik M, Berelowitz M, Dhillon AP, Thomson MA, Harvey P, Valentine A, Davies SE, Walker-Smith JA. Ileal lymphoid nodular hyperplasia, non-specific colitis and pervasive developmental disorder in children. *The Lancet*. 1998;351:637-641. [retracted]

[3] Rout M. (2009, April 1). Vioxx maker Merck and Co drew up doctor hit list. Retrieved from http://aftermathnews.wordpress.com/2009/04/27/vioxx-maker-merck-and-co-drew-up-doctor-hit-list/

[4] Stone M. (2010, February 22). Toyota recall investigation uncovers documents = saving money better than saving lives. examiner.com. Retrieved from: http://www.examiner.com/examiner/x-19632-Salt-Lake-City-Headlines-Examiner~y2010m2d22-Toyota-recall-investigation-uncovers-documents--saving-money-better-than-savings-lives.

[5] McIntyre D. (2010, February 12). Daily Finance. Toyota Used Ex-Regulators to Help Kill Probes. Retrieved from: http://www.dailyfinance.com/story/company-news/toyota-used-ex-regulators-to-help-kill-probes/19355607/

[6] Freed G, Clark S, Butchart A, Singer D, Davis, M. Parental Vaccine Safety Concerns in 2009. *Pediatrics*. 2010;125(4);654-659. Retrieved from: http://pediatrics.aappublications.org/cgi/reprint/peds.2009-1962v1.

[7] Bill and Melinda Gates Foundation. (2010, January 29). Bill and Melinda Gates Pledge $10 Billion in Call for Decade of Vaccines.
Retrieved from http://www.gatesfoundation.org/press-releases/Pages/decade-of-vaccines-wec-announcement-100129.aspx.

[8] Age of Autism. (2009, February 27). Why is the Media Ignoring the Bailey Banks Autism Vaccine Decision? Retrieved from http://www.ageofautism.com/2009/02/why-is-the-mediaignoring-the-bailey-banks-autism-vaccine-decision.html.

See also Bailey Banks, by his father Kenneth Banks vs. Secretary of the Department of Health and Human Services. United States Court of Federal Claims. 20 July 2007.

Retrieved from http://www.uscfc.uscourts.gov/sites/default/files/Abell.BANKS.02-0738V.pdf

[9] Attkisson S. (2008, June 19). Vaccine Watch. CBS News Investigates: Primary Source. Retrieved from http://www.cbsnews.com/8301-501263_162-4194102-501263.html.
See also Afterword, "Ethics, Evidence, and the Death of Medicine."

CHAPTER ONE

That Paper

On February 28, 1998, twelve colleagues and I published a case series paper in *The Lancet*, a respected medical journal, as an "Early Report."[1] The paper described the clinical findings in 12 children with an autistic spectrum disorder (ASD) occurring in association with a mild-to-moderate inflammation of the large intestine (colitis). This was accompanied by swelling of the lymph glands in the intestinal lining (lymphoid nodular hyperplasia), predominantly in the last part of the small intestine (terminal ileum). Contemporaneously, parents of 9 children associated onset of symptoms with measles, mumps, and rubella (MMR) vaccine exposure, 8 of whom were reported on in the original paper (see also Child PH's story on following page). The significance of these findings has been overshadowed by misunderstanding, misrepresentation, and a concerted, systematic effort to discredit the work. This effort, and specifically the complaint of a freelance journalist and an intense political desire to subvert enquiry into issues of vaccine safety and legal redress for vaccine damage, culminated in the longest running and most expensive fitness to practice case ever to come before the United Kingdom's medical regulator, the General Medical Council. At this point, the guilty verdict is in. Now, and only now, with all of the contemporaneous documentation available, is it timely to review both the original paper and its legacy.

Background
From the late 1980s, my team at the Royal Free Hospital School of Medicine, the Inflammatory Bowel Disease Study Group, published extensively on possible causes and mechanisms of inflammatory bowel disease (e.g., Crohn's disease). This involved examination of a possible causal role for measles and measles vaccine. In May 1995, parents started contacting me with the story that their normally developing child had regressed into autism or an autism-like state, with onset in the majority of cases soon after MMR vaccine. At around the same time, the children had developed chronic gastrointestinal (GI) symptoms similar to those described by Dr. Lenny Gonzalez in the July 2009 edition of *The Autism File*.[2] Despite what were often debilitating intestinal symptoms, many indicative of abdominal

pain, few of these children had undergone physical examination, let alone been investigated. Mention of the MMR vaccine had often alienated parents further from their child's health care providers. Many doctors attributed the onset of symptoms to coincidence and were content to leave it at that. Conversely, at the Royal Free a systematic plan of clinical care and research was designed in order to help affected children.

Child PH's* story, as originally told by his mother, did not cite MMR as the culprit. Eighteen months of normal development was followed by regression, giving rise to what several doctors labeled "secondary autism." Loss of developmental milestones was accompanied by loss of coordination (he could no longer throw and catch a ball), his gait became, "awkward and stiff like an old man," and he could no longer go from sitting to standing unaided. He lost the 20 words that he had gained and developed secondary fecal incontinence. At 18 months of age, severe episodes of abdominal pain started that were associated with screaming and drawing his knees to his chest. He developed a pattern of chronic loose bowel motions with undigested food from 2 years of age. He went from the 97th centile for weight at 1 year of age to the 50th by age 2. His diet went from being varied to very restricted, consisting of refined carbohydrates and at least ten 200 ml cartons of orange-flavored drink per day.

What Child PH's mother did not tell us in 1996 was that, contemporaneously, **she too had linked her son's problems to MMR vaccine**. Our description of this child in *The Lancet* faithfully reiterated the onset of symptoms following an episode of otitis media as his mother had reported but made no mention of the MMR. The reason for this discordance in the narrative provides a valuable lesson: the reaction of successive doctors to the suggestion that MMR might have been involved ranged from patronizingly dismissive to outright hostile. Mentioning the vaccine was beginning to negatively impact their ability to get help for their son. By the time they came to the Royal Free Hospital, the father had urged his wife not to mention the MMR again in order to avoid discrimination by doctors who considered her to be crazy.

So it was that a potentially important element of the clinical history in this child had been corrupted by the arrogance of those who "knew better."

*Initials have been changed.

Study design

The Lancet paper – the first in a series of related papers – is a **case series**: This is stated explicitly in the first line of the paper: "…a consecutive series of children with chronic entero-colitis and regressive developmental disorder."[1] A typical example of how basic epidemiological textbooks define and describe a case series is found in Hennekens and Buring:[3]

> Case series studies **describe** the experience of a single patient or a **group of patients** with a **similar diagnosis**. These types of study, in which typically an astute clinician identifies **an unusual feature of a disease** or a patient's history, may lead to **formulation of a new hypothesis**… At that time an analytic study (most frequently using a case-control approach), can [then] be done to investigate possible causal factors.

The crucial design feature that differentiates the **case series** from other designs is its lack of requirement to select participants on the basis of either the exposure (e.g., MMR) or the outcome of interest (e.g., autism). A case series does not require – and should not employ – strict inclusion or exclusion criteria. Rather, it should function to observe similar presentations in groups of patients that appear to share other common features in order to raise hypotheses that later may be tested in the appropriate study design framework (e.g., a **case-control** study).

The Lancet paper does exactly what is required of a case series. It states immediately what the report sets out to do: no particular developmental disorder was stated, no particular features or timing of onset were required, no particular initial exposure was necessary, no specific outcome was predicted, and no causal association was claimed.

Of note, we have been criticized for not having controls in the study; that is, developmentally normal children included for the purpose of comparison. While controls are not usually part of a case series, we went beyond what would normally be required and *did* include comparison groups – 19 age-matched children (5 for microscopic examination of tissues and 14 for measurement of urinary methylmalonic acid [MMA]). This would have been evident upon a proper reading of the paper.

Finally, Hennekens and Buring make the crucial point that the purpose of a case series is to **generate new hypotheses** about potential causation. It is **not** designed to investigate possible causality. The Lancet paper was hypothesis generating; it stimulated a series of subsequent papers – rarely if ever acknowledged by critics – that confirmed and characterized the bowel disease as novel, relatively frequent, and potentially treatable and tested ideas about causation.[4] Among the critics there has been some confusion on this point, which is evident, for example, in a widely quoted analysis of the paper by Professor Trisha Greenhalgh[5] that raises and attempts to answer a series of questions, including:

Was the research hypothesis clearly stated?

She observes, "The paper does not state a research hypothesis at all." This is quite true. Case series studies are neither required nor expected to do so. Having established that there was no hypothesis, Professor Greenhalgh goes on to pose the ridiculous question:

Was this design an appropriate way to test the research hypothesis?

She concludes that the study design was not an appropriate way to test "the research hypothesis." However, since she has already identified the fact that no hypothesis was stated, she rather begs the question as to which hypothesis the study was not designed to test. It soon becomes clear that it was *her* hypothesis that the study did not test. Her conclusion that "the study design was incapable of proving the [MMR] link one way or the other" is, of course, entirely accurate as we had already indicated in the paper on page 641, paragraph 2, lines 1 and 2:[1]

> We did not prove an association between measles, mumps and rubella vaccine and the syndrome described. . . .

and paragraph 5, lines 4-6:

> Further investigations are needed to examine this syndrome and its possible relation to the vaccine.

Professor Greenhalgh ventures even further off course when she asks:

Were the study's conclusions supported by the data?

It is not clear whether Professor Greenhalgh is referring to the *authors'* conclusions – i.e., that the data do not demonstrate a causal link between the disorder and MMR exposure and that further research is required, or whether she is asking if the data support the hypothesis that she has eroneously imputed to the study authors. In the former case, the data clearly support our conclusions. Not surprisingly, they do not support Professor Greenhalgh's contrived hypothesis – that MMR causes the syndrome described.

She continues:

If the answer to [the question above] is "no," would a more robust study design have been practically possible to test the study's main hypothesis?

Continuing to build an argument on a hypothesis of her own construction, Professor Greenhalgh answers her question with a resounding "yes." That she does appear satisfied, on the basis of what can only be described as a complete misunderstanding of *The Lancet* study's design, is cause for concern. In turn, the failure of the Department of Health (whose website directed people via the National Health Service Executive to her analysis) to appreciate the potential impact of this deeply flawed document on the perceptions of many thousands of worried parents is alarming.

Notwithstanding Professor Greenhalgh's follies, one should never underestimate the importance of the case series as a starting point for medical discovery. It is the tried and tested mode of the description of human disease syndromes, including Kanner's autism, Asperger's syndrome, and Heller's disease (disintegrative disorder). One final word on the matter endorses this perspective:

> *Clinical situations in which a case report or case series is an appropriate type of study include the following: a doctor notices that two babies born in his hospital have absent limbs (phocomelia). Both mothers had taken a new drug (thalidomide) in early pregnancy. The doctor wishes to alert his colleagues worldwide to the possibility of drug related damage as quickly as possible (McBride, in The Lancet 1961). Anyone who thinks 'quick and dirty' case reports are never scientifically justified should remember this example.*

And the source of this invaluable piece of advice? Dr. Trisha Greenhalgh, author of "How to Read a Paper."[6]

"Coincidence"

Coincidence – often the first resort of skeptical physicians – refers, in this context, to the chance occurrence of autistic symptoms being identified in the second year of life, at around the same time as MMR is given. Regularly advanced as an explanation for the parents' story, coincidence is a conclusion of last resort – one that should be arrived at only after diagnostic due diligence has excluded alternative causes for neurological deterioration in a child. Meticulous attention should be paid to the parental history, and the practice of claiming coincidence without first excluding possible causes has no place in clinical medicine. Where an infection such as herpes simplex or Epstein-Barr virus (mono) has preceded autistic regression, the medical literature shows that extensive testing has been undertaken, the cause identified, and the child treated accordingly.[7] In contrast, when MMR vaccination has preceded autistic regression, little, if any, attempt has been made to investigate children appropriately. The case of Bailey Banks is one of those rare instances where this has been done and for whom the United States vaccine court ruled that MMR caused his ASD.[8] Bailey's MRI, performed 16 days post-MMR for encephalopathy, revealed abnormalities of brain myelin consistent with acute disseminated encephalomyelitis (ADEM), an autoimmune brain inflammation that can follow measles or a measles vaccine. The lesson is that every attempt should be made to evaluate children during the course of their regression since, as in the case of ADEM, abnormalities of brain myelin may be transient and not evident on an MRI performed 2 years after exposure. The fact that the parents of *The Lancet* children described loss of fecal and/or urinary continence in four cases and ataxia (clumsiness) in at least six – the latter being a reported adverse reaction to MMR vaccine – is more than enough indication for thorough neurological workup. The history of regression with loss of acquired skills in a previously normal or near-normal child should ring alarm bells and initiate a systematic approach to differential diagnosis. It was with this in mind that Professor Walker-Smith, one of the world's leading pediatric gastroenterologists and senior author of *The Lancet* paper, wrote in 1997:

[These children] *have not had the level of investigation which we would regard as adequate for a child presenting with such a devastating condition.*[9]

Despite evident neurological symptoms, despite the proximity of onset to a viral exposure, and despite additional physical symptoms such as pain and diarrhea, a diagnosis of autism trumped the need for anything but minimal investigation by "mainstream" autism practitioners for the majority of these children.

Coincidence and rechallenge

Where a child with regressive autism has received more than one dose of a measles-containing vaccine (MCV), exacerbation of existing symptoms and/or recurrence of transient symptoms associated with the first dose is frequently reported. Properly documented, the Institute of Medicine's Vaccine Safety Committee accepts the "rechallenge" effect as evidence of causation.[10] In order to examine this in the setting of MMR and *autistic enterocolitis* and to overcome the concern about parental recall of events that may have occurred many years before, we conducted a study comparing the severity of intestinal inflammation between children once-vaccinated and those twice-vaccinated with an MCV. Our hypothesis was that the disease should be more severe in those exposed twice if the disease were caused by the vaccine.[11] There was a significantly higher prevalence of active chronic colitis (involving pus-forming cells) in those children given an MMR or measles and rubella (MR) booster compared with those receiving only one dose, supporting a causal association. This apparent rechallenge effect is currently being examined in a large population of US children to see if the finding is reproducible.

Rechallenge with a measles vaccine

Child RT* was monitored closely in his first year due to wide bridging of his nose. He was discharged from follow-up as developmentally and physically normal by 15 months of age. He later received a single measles vaccine following which he stopped "cruising" around furniture and regressed to crawling. His learning plateaued and, by 20 months, he had lost words; soon thereafter, he stopped talking altogether. General ill health developed in his second year with ear, chest, and throat infections, and diarrhea with abdominal pain. According to his mother's story, 2 weeks after an MMR vaccine, at 4.5 years of age, he "disappeared" and "lost all skills and communication." While at 10 months of age he had been able to build a tower of bricks, his play skills declined to the point that, "now he [was] lost as to what to do with them." In addition, he became clumsy, started head banging, and developed repetitive behaviors. He lost his self-help skills; for example, before the MMR booster he could feed himself with a spoon, afterwards he could no longer even hold a cup.

The history of Child RT's GI problems is also instructive. His records state: "The diarrhoea became a problem at between 1-1½ years of age [after his single measles vaccine]... it generally contains undigested food. His diarrhea became significantly worse from 4½ years of age [after his MMR]..." Failure to thrive, a cardinal sign of pediatric inflammatory bowel disease, was evident from the GP's records; he was reported to be "dropping off centile charts." This failure to thrive continued and took another downturn at the same time that his diarrhea worsened, when he was noted to have dropped from the 9th to the 2nd centile for weight.

Further examination of MMR rechallenge is currently under way.

*Initials have been changed.

Diligent science

The quest for precision can become a hostage to fortune, as the microscopic analysis of *The Lancet* children's tissues was to prove. There are few people in the world with Professor Walker-Smith's knowledge of the microscopic appearances of inflammatory disease of the intestine in children. So it was that, in the absence of a pediatric pathologist expert in this field at the Royal Free, Professor Walker-Smith conducted a weekly review of his patients' tissues and identified the fact that disease was being missed in some children. In order to reduce this risk and to standardize the reporting of the ASD children's biopsies, all tissues were subsequently examined by a single senior pathologist with expertise in bowel disease. His findings were recorded on a specially designed chart to document specific features of tissue damage.[12] This record formed the basis of what was subsequently reported in *The Lancet*. Few case series go to this level of precision.

In the hands of someone determined to discredit the work, however, discrepancies between the routine clinical report (which may have come, for example, from a pathologist with an interest in brain disease or gynecological pathology) and the standardized expert analysis were falsely reported in the national media as "fixing" of the data. I was specifically accused of this, although I had no part in scoring the reviews. It is notable that despite 5 years of investigation by the GMC, no charge of scientific fraud has been made against any of the defendants. The allegation of fraud was made by the same freelance journalist who had actually also initiated the GMC enquiry, continuing his litany of false allegations. There is no evidence at all that the data had been "fixed" as was alleged, and the newspaper in question has failed to produce any, despite a request to do so from the Press Complaints Commission. Paradoxically, the price paid for diligent science has been a headline proclaiming fraud. In my opinion, the intended goal – to reinforce the false belief that the work is discredited – has been achieved.

The damage done

The damage done to my reputation and to that of my colleagues as well as the personal price for pursuing a valid scientific question while putting the patients' interests above all others is trivial compared with the impact of these falsehoods on the children's access to appropriate and necessary care. My experience serves as a cynical example to discourage others. As a consequence, many physicians in the United Kingdom and United States will not risk providing the care that is due to these children. There is a pervasive and openly stated bias against funding and publication of this work, and I have been excluded from presenting at meetings on the instructions of the sponsoring pharmaceutical company. This episode in medical history has been an effective exercise in public relations and selling newspapers. But it will fail – it will fail because nature cannot be deceived.

It has always been a privilege working on behalf of children with autism and their families. It is my hope that before too long the tide will turn and that, in addition, my teacher and mentor Professor Sir Stanley Peart, FRS, will come to realize that I have never forsaken his instruction.

Myths

The Lancet paper was funded by the Legal Aid Board (LAB)[13]

False – Not one penny of LAB money was spent on *The Lancet* paper. A LAB grant was provided for a separate viral detection study. This latter study, completed in 1999, does disclose the source of funding. *The Lancet* paper had been submitted for publication before the LAB grant was even available to be spent.

My involvement as a medical expert was kept "secret"[14]

False – at least 1 year before publication, I informed my senior coauthors,[15] the head of the department, the dean of the medical school,[16] and the CEO of the hospital. This fact was also reported in the national press 15 months prior to publication.[17]

Children were "sourced" by lawyers to sue vaccine manufacturers[14]

False – Children were referred, evaluated, and investigated on the basis of their clinical symptoms alone, following referral from the child's physician.[18]

Children were litigants[19]

False – at the time of their referral to the Royal Free, the time material to their inclusion in *The Lancet* paper, none of the children were litigants.

I had an undisclosed conflict of interest[20]

False – *The Lancet*'s disclosure policy at that time was followed to the letter. Documentary evidence confirms that the editorial staff of *The Lancet* was fully aware that I was working as an expert on MMR litigation well in advance of the paper's publication.[21]

Did not have ethics committee (EC) approval[14]

False – The research element of the paper that required such an approval, detailed systematic analysis of children's intestinal biopsies, was covered by the necessary EC approval.[22]

I "fixed" data and misreported clinical findings[23]

False – There is absolutely no basis in fact for this claim and it has been exposed as false.[24]

Findings have not been independently replicated[21]

False – The key findings of lymphoid nodular hyperplasia (LNH) and colitis in ASD children have been independently confirmed in five different countries.[25]

Has been retracted by most of the authors[26]

False – 11 of 13 authors issued a retraction of the interpretation that MMR is a possible trigger for syndrome described. This remains a possibility and a possibility cannot be retracted.

The work is discredited[27]

False – Those attemping to discredit the work have relied upon the myths above. The findings described in the paper are novel and important.[4]

The legacy of *The Lancet* paper

The first demonstration of intestinal pathology in ASD
GI symptoms are common in children with autism, and these symptoms are frequently associated with intestinal inflammation.
Treatment of GI inflammation may lead to symptomatic improvement in both GI and behavioral symptoms.[28]

The first demonstration of abnormal vitamin B12 metabolism in ASD
Now the subject of major clinical and research activities in autism, ranging from study of genetic differences in B12/folate metabolism to treatment with active forms of B12.

The first study to report a rechallenge effect of a measles containing vaccine (MCV)
Follow-up indicates that intestinal inflammation is significantly worse in rechallenge ASD children than children receiving only one MCV.[11]

First study to seek evidence of a mitochondrial disorder by measurement of lactate:pyruvate in cerebrospinal fluid
"Mito" disorders appear to be common in ASD children and may be acquired. The US government conceded that vaccines triggered autism in Hannah Poling, a child with "mito" disorder.[29]

Did they read the paper?

Ari Brown, MD. Spokesperson for the American Academy of Pediatrics and the Immunization Action Coalition

"This flawed study concluded that the rise in autism was related to giving the combination vaccine of measles-mumps-rubella (MMR)."[30]

Professor Sir Michael Rutter, FRS. Expert prosecution witness GMC, expert witness on behalf of MMR vaccine manufacturers

"Publication of a study claiming a casual relationship between measles, mumps and rubella (MMR) vaccine and autism spectrum disorders (ASD) sparked a heated debate..."[31]

Professor Eric Fombonne. Expert witness on behalf of MMR vaccine manufacturers

"Recent reports claim to have identified another variant of autism (called 'autistic enterocolitis') in children referred to a gastroenterology department. The hypothesis has involved 3 separate claims: 1) that a new phenotype of autism associated with developmental regression and gastro-intestinal symptoms has emerged as a consequence of measles-mumps-rubella vaccination..."[32]

Endnotes

[1] Wakefield A, et al. Ileal lymphoid nodular hyperplasia, non-specific colitis and pervasive developmental disorder in children. *The Lancet* 1998;351:637-641. [retracted]

[2] Gonzalez L. Gastrointestinal Pathology in Autism Spectrum Disorders: the Venezuelan Experience. *The Autism File.* 2009;32:34-37.

[3] Hennekens C, Buring, J. (1987) *Epidemiology in Medicine.* Mayrent, SL (Ed.), Philadelphia, PA: Lippincott, Williams and Wilkins.

[4] Horvath K, et al. High prevalence of gastrointestinal symptoms in children with autistic spectrum disorder (ASD). *J Pediatr Gastroenterol Nutr* 2000, 31:S174.

Melmed R, et al. Metabolic markers and gastrointestinal symptoms in children with autism and related disorders. *J Pediatr Gastroenterol Nutr* 2000, 31:S31–S32.

Horvath K, Perman J. Autistic disorder and gastrointestinal disease. *Current Opinion in Pediatrics* 2002;14:583–587.

Furlano R, et al. Quantitative immunohistochemistry shows colonic epithelial pathology and γδ-T cell infiltration in autistic enterocolitis. *J Pediatrics* 2001;138:366-372.

Torrente F, et al. Enteropathy with T cell infiltration and epithelial IgG deposition in autism. *Molecular Psychiatry.* 2002;7:375-382.

Torrente F, et al. Focal-enhanced gastritis in regressive autism with features distinct from Crohn's and helicobacter pylori gastritis. *Am. J. Gastroenterol.* 2004;4:598-605.

Ashwood P, et al. Intestinal lymphocyte populations in children with regressive autism: Evidence for extensive mucosal immunopathology. *J. Clin. Immunol.* 2003;23:504-517.

Ashwood P, et al. Spontaneous mucosal lymphocyte cytokine profiles in children with regressive autism and gastrointestinal symptoms: Mucosal immune activation and reduced counter regulatory interleukin-10. *Journal of Clinical Immunology.* 2004:24:664-673.

Wakefield A. Entero-colonic encephalopathy, autism and opioid receptor ligands. *Alimentary Pharmacology & Therapeutics.* 2002;16:663-674.

Uhlmann V, et al. Potential viral pathogenic mechanism for new variant inflammatory bowel disease. *Molecular Pathology* 2002;55:84-90.

Sabra A, et al. Ileal-lymphoid-nodular hyperplasia, non-specific colitis and pervasive developmental disorder in children. *The Lancet,* 1998;352:234-235.

Sabra A, et al. Linkage of ileal-lymphoid-nodular hyperplasia (ILNH), food allergy and CNS developmental: evidence for a non-IgE association. *Ann Allergy Asthma Immunol,* 1999;82:8.

Valicenti-McDermott M, et al. Frequency of gastrointestinal symptoms in children with autistic spectrum disorders and association with family history of autoimmune disease. *Developmental and Behavioral Pediatrics.* 2006;27:128-136.

Richler J, Luyster, R, Risi S, Hsu W, Dawson G, Bernier, R, et al. Is there a 'regressive phenotype' of autistic spectrum disorder associated with the measles-mumps-rubella vaccine? A CPEA study. *Autism Dev Dis* 2006, 36:299-316.

Sandler R. Short-term benefit from oral vancomycin treatment of regressive-onset autism. *J Child Neurol.* 2000;15:429-435.

Parracho H. Differences between the gut flora of children with autistic spectrum disorders and that of healthy children. *Journal of Medical Microbiology.* 2005;54:987-991.

[5] Greenhalgh T. A critical appraisal of the Wakefield et al paper. Retrieved from http://briandeer.com/mmr/lancet-greenhalgh.htm

[6] Greenhalgh T. How to Read a Paper. *BMJ* 2001;326:106-106.

[7] DeLong R, et al. Acquired reversible autistic syndrome in acute encephalopathic illness in children. *Child Neurology.* 1981;38:191-194.

Gillberg C. Brief report: onset at age 14 of a typical autistic syndrome. A case report of a girl with herpes simplex encephalitis. *J Aut Dev Dis.* 1986;16:369-375.

Shenoy S, et al. Response to steroid therapy in autism secondary to autoimmune lympho-proliferative syndrome *J Pediatrics.* 2000;136:682-687.

[8] *Age of Autism.* (2009, February 27). Why is the Media Ignoring the Bailey Banks Autism Vaccine Decision? Retrieved from http://www.ageofautism.com/2009/02/why-is-the-media-ignoring-the-bailey-banks-autism-vaccine-decision.html

[9] Correspondence: Walker-Smith JA to Pegg M. (Chairman Ethical Practices Committee). November 11, 1996.

[10] Stratton K, et al. (1994). *Adverse Events Associated with Childhood Vaccines: Evidence Bearing on Causality.* Washington, D.C.: National Academies Press.

[11] Wakefield, A. Gastrointestinal co-morbidity, autistic regression and measles-containing vaccines: positive re-challenge and biological gradient effects. *Medical Veritas* 2006;3:796-802.

[12] Wakefield A. Enterocolitis in children with developmental disorder. *American Journal of Gastroenterology* 2000;95:2285-2295.

Wakefield A. Autistic enterocolitis: Is it a histological entity? *Histopathology* 2006;50:380-384.

[13] Allegation by Brian Deer to *The Lancet* editor Richard Horton, February 2004 and January 2008. General Certificate of School Education (GCSE) Biology exam (higher tier). Assessment and Qualifications Alliance. http://www.aqa.org.uk/ (home page). See also Chapter 13, "Poisoning Young Minds" in this book.

[14] *Revealed: MMR Research Scandal Brian Deer.* (2004, February 22). *The Sunday Times.*

[15] Correspondence between Dr. Wakefield and Professor Walker-Smith, February 3, 1997 and February 20, 1997.

[16] Correspondence between Dr. Wakefield and Professor AJ Zuckerman, March 24, 1997.

[17] Langdon-Down G. (1996, November 27). "Law: A shot in the Dark." *The Independent.* Page 25.

[18] Statement of Walker-Smith J. *The Lancet* 2004;363:822-823.

[19] *The Sunday Times.* February 2004 and January 2008. General Certificate of School Education (GCSE) Biology exam (higher tier). Assessment and Qualifications Alliance.

http://www.aqa.org.uk/ (home page). See also Chapter 13, "Poisoning Young Minds" in this book.

[20] *Revealed: MMR Research Scandal Brian Deer.* (2004, February 22). *The Sunday Times.* Also, Horton R, A statement by the editors of *The Lancet. The Lancet* 2004;363:820-821.

[21] Moody J. Complaint to GMC vs Horton R., Zuckerman A., Pegg M., and Salisbury D. (complaint filed and pending).

[22] Carroll, M. to Walker-Smith, J. Ethical Practices Committee approval 162/95. Date of approval September 5, 1995.

[23] Deer B. (2009, February 8) MMR doctor Andrew Wakefield fixed data on autism. *The Sunday Times.*

[24] Complaint to Press Complaints Commission. Wakefield vs Deer and *The Sunday Times.* (see www.cryshame.org).

[25] In addition to the UK: Gonzalez L, et al. Endoscopic and Histological Characteristics of the Digestive Mucosa in Autistic Children with gastro-Intestinal Symptoms. *Arch Venez Pueric Pediatr,* 2005;69:19-25. And Balzola F, et al. Panenteric IBD-like disease in a patient with regressive autism shown for the first time by wireless capsule enteroscopy: Another piece in the jig-saw of the gut-brain syndrome? *American Journal of Gastroenterology,* 2005. 100(4):979-981.

Krigsman A, et al. http://www.cevs.ucdavis.edu/Cofred/Public/Aca/WebSec. cfm?confid=238&webid=1245 (last accessed June 2007) [no longer available; full paper now published below as:

Galiatsatos P, Gologan A, Lamoureux E. Autistic enterocolitis: fact or fiction. *Canadian Journal of Gastroenterology.* 2009;23:95-98.

Krigsman A, Boris M, Goldblatt A, Stott C. Clinical Presentation and Histologic Findings at Ileocolonoscopy in Children with Autistic Spectrum Disorder and Chronic Gastrointestinal Symptoms. *Autism Insights.* 2009;1:1–11.

Chen B, Girgis S, El-Matary W. Childhood autism and eosinophilic colitis. *Digestion.* 2010;81:127-9. Epub 2010 Jan 9].

[26] Evidence of Horton R, to the General Medical Council; statement of Horton R, *The Lancet* 2004;363:820-821.

[27] briandeer.com. Six year media investigation forces the *Lancet* retraction of fraudulent research. Retrieved from http://briandeer.com/mmr/lancet-retraction.htm

[28] Walker-Smith J, et al. Ileo-caecal lymphoid nodular hyperplasia, ileo-colitis with regressive behavioural disorder and food intolerance: a case study. *J. Paediatric gastroenterology and Nutrition.* 1997;25:Suppl 48:A31.

Balzola F, et al. Beneficial behavioural effects of IBD therapy and gluten/casein-free diet in an Italian cohort of patients with autistic enterocolitis followed over one year. *Gastroenterology:*2008;4:S1364.

[29] Poling J, Poling T. (2008, April 5). Vaccines, autism and our daughter Hannah. *The New York Times.*

Poling J, et al. Developmental regression and mitochondrial dysfunction in a child with autism. *J Child Neurol,* 2006;21(2):170–2.

Oliveira G, et al. Epidemiology of autism spectrum disorder in Portugal: Prevalence, clinical characterization, and medical conditions. *Dev Med Child Neurol.* 2007;49(10):726–33.

Elliot H, et al. Pathogenic mitochondrial DNA mutations are common in the general population. *Am J Human Genetics* 2008;83:254–60.

Filipek P, et al. Mitochondrial dysfunction in autistic patients with 15q inverted duplication. *Ann Neurol,* 2003; 53: 801–4.

[30] Brown A, Fields D. (2005). *Baby 411.* Boulder, CO: Windsor Peak Press.

[31] Honda H, Shimizu Y, Rutter M. No effect of MMR withdrawal on the incidence of autism: a total population study. *J Child Psychol Psychiatry,* 2005;46(6):572–9.

[32] Fombonne E, Chakrabarti S. No evidence for a new variant of measles-mumps-rubella-induced autism. *Pediatrics* 2001;108:4. The 1998 paper in *The Lancet* makes no reference to autistic enterocolitis and makes no claims relating to a new variant *autism.* It doesn't *claim* that the new phenotype is a consequence of MMR. Wakefield A, et al., 2000, doesn't mention MMR or vaccination at all.

CHAPTER TWO

The Children

This chapter describes the clinical presentation of the first children with autism spectrum disorder (ASD) and intestinal symptoms of unknown origin who were seen at the Royal Free Hospital. In a less compromised world, these presentations (and those in many thousands more children worldwide) and the pattern that emerged from the commonalities in their symptoms and clinical findings should have initiated a cascade of urgent clinical research that would have led through an iterative process to discovery – discovery of cause, treatment, and prevention. Sadly, this has not been the case.

For now, let's start with the children. In May 1995, I received the sentinel call from Rosemary Kessick (in accordance with the GMC's anonymous coding, she is the mother of Child 2). Intelligent and articulate, Rosemary's motive was to improve her son's well-being rather than to apportion blame. She was of the considered conviction that her child's regression into autism, his long-standing diarrhea and food intolerances, and the simultaneous fluctuations in behavioral and intestinal symptoms meant that they were linked. Moreover, she had come to the prescient conclusions that an abnormality of vitamin B12 might somehow be involved and that this whole process had been triggered by his MMR vaccine. Rosemary was aware of many children with a similar story.

It was obvious that whatever else Child 2 needed, his gastrointestinal (GI) symptoms required investigation. I recommended that she seek a referral from her son's doctor to John Walker-Smith who was, at that time, a professor of pediatric gastroenterology at St. Bartholomew's Hospital, within the walls of the old City of London. In autumn 1995, with St. Bartholomew's under threat of closure, Walker-Smith and his team transferred to the Royal Free Hospital where children with developmental disorders and intestinal issues were referred to his care in increasing numbers, adding a physically and emotionally demanding clinical commitment to what was already the busiest pediatric gastroenterology service in the UK. In many cases, the parents made initial contact with me, and after listening to their stories, if it transpired that their child had GI problems, I would recommend that they seek an appointment with

Walker-Smith. I offered to talk to the child's doctor if further information was required on what it was that we considered might be the link between the intestine and the neurological injury in this population of children. The doctor, so informed, was in a position to weigh the merits of making a clinical referral. As will be discussed, this process, however benign and helpful it might have been, was to be transmuted into something sinister at the GMC hearing.

In July 1996, it was by virtue of a quirk of timing — a mix-up with a school holiday — that the first patient, Rosemary's son, was not the first of these children to undergo colonoscopy. Another young boy (Child 1) was to be the first child investigated by Walker-Smith and his team. Child 1 had developed normally to 18 months of age and regressed soon after MMR with a clearly delineated onset with loss of words, comprehension, and social interaction plus secondary fecal and urinary incontinence. In his history, the passage of blood and undigested food in his feces provided more than enough indication for ileocolonoscopy. I was away at a conference during his admission and visited the department of pediatric gastroenterology with some trepidation upon my return. Would there be a record of some form of intestinal inflammation in this child that might be amenable to treatment and symptomatic relief?

In the UK, it is routine practice for all patients to have a *discharge summary* prepared soon after they leave the hospital. This document summarizes the patient's stay in the hospital, outlining findings, treatment recommendations, etc., and is intended to keep the patient's family doctor and other doctors involved in the patient's care fully up-to-date with their patient. Child 1's discharge summary — prepared by a junior doctor — stated that other than lymphoid nodular hyperplasia (LNH) no abnormality was found in his colon. I read this with a mixture of surprise and disappointment; had the wrong call been made, leaving no new avenues of potential benefit for this child? I checked the pathology report against the detailed clinical records documented at the time of colonoscopy. They described a definite ulcer in the rectum, the lowest part of the large intestine. When I read the report of the microscopic examination of his intestinal biopsies, I saw that the pathologist had described chronic active inflammation — not definitively Crohn's disease or ulcerative colitis — but clear evidence of disease. In addition, levels of digestive enzymes measured in samples taken from his upper intestine were uniformly low, providing an explanation for the appearance of undigested food in his stool. After alerting Walker-Smith to this important discrepancy, he had the discharge summary amended to reflect the facts. Child 1 was put on anti-inflammatory medication (Salazopyrin[6]) of the sort that is used routinely to treat inflammatory bowel disease. He responded beyond our expectations. Six months later he was discharged from the clinic. The entry in his records reads:

> ...*definite improvement, both in gastrointestinal symptoms and cognition/ communication/behaviors.*

William (Child 2) was admitted to the hospital in September 1996. His story was not the course of typical autism, but one of progressive deterioration that had been documented by experts from several different institutions. One had stated:

> ...*sadly both the rating scale scores and the repeat assessments demonstrate that William has lost skills over the last 3 years. This pattern of ongoing regression is not one which is normally observed in children with autism even among the group who have an early loss of skills in the latter half of the 2nd year. The expected course for children with autism is one of continuing progress... in the light of this situation it now seems important to investigate William for the full range of neurodegenerative conditions.*

William had been seen previously by a pediatric neurologist at Great Ormond Street Hospital, one of the UK's foremost children's hospitals. Having seen him, the pediatric neurologist wrote to the referring physician:

> *Thank you for letting me see this 8-year-old boy who now has features of a child with classic infantile autism. What is unusual is that there have been three episodes of regression each preceded by some months of increased activity and misery. Following each episode of regression he has never regained the skills lost... I am afraid I do not recognize this as a defined neurometabolic or immunological disorder. However I do think reinvestigation is necessary... I would suggest the following investigation: MRI,[1] EEG,[2] metabolic investigations, detailed immunological investigations of both T and B cell function and immunological consultation, and gastrointestinal consultation.*

In the interim, as part of Rosemary's strategy of leaving no stone unturned, she had anticipated the need for further input into William's intestinal symptoms and had taken him to see an adult gastroenterologist in Cambridge, an expert in the use of nutrition and the manipulation of intestinal bacteria to treat intestinal inflammation. He prescribed probiotics — good bacteria, which apparently had improved William's gastrointestinal symptoms. At the same time, this doctor had identified a raised inflammatory marker in William's blood, namely the erythrocyte sedimentation rate (sed rate or ESR) at 40mm/hr[3] when the normal rate should be 0-15mm/hr. The GMC's prosecution witness was later to interpret William's symptomatic improvement on probiotics as a contraindication to him undergoing colonoscopy. On the contrary, this positive beneficial response to bowel treatment combined with his high sed rate was confirmation of an intestinal disease until proven otherwise.

This was confirmed at colonoscopy where one definite ulcer was seen, and the colon and the ileum showed marked swelling of the intestinal lymph glands (referred to earlier as lymphoid nodular hyperplasia or LNH). Microscopic examination of the intestinal biopsies showed chronic active inflammation of the bowel lining with the presence of pus-forming cells (neutrophils) in the mucus-producing glands of the colon (cryptitis) with architectural damage to the crypts. These are findings that are seen commonly in inflammatory bowel disease and were evident in many of the autistic children. The patchy distribution of this inflammation and the involvement of the terminal ileum were considered to be consistent with a diagnosis of Crohn's disease. On the basis of this diagnosis, William was entered into a clinical trial of a special nutritional formula (polymeric diet). He made a dramatic response both from the bowel and behavioral perspective. I remember his delighted mother telling us that her son had started laughing and playing again, something that he had not done for years. So impressive was William's case that the findings were presented to an international meeting of pediatric gastroenterologists by Walker-Smith in 1997.[4]

And so the pattern continued: Child 3's history was of normal development followed by sudden changes in behavior just 2 days after MMR vaccination at 14 months, when he started head-banging accompanied by fever and rash. At 15 months of age he underwent a dramatic deterioration in behavior, with hand flapping (a very common feature of autism), aggression, and deterioration in speech. By the time he was 2 years old, he could no longer speak. From the very outset, his mother was convinced of the association between her child's deterioration and MMR vaccination. His bowel problems started with diarrhea and progressed to chronic laxative-dependent constipation, pain, and the passage of blood in his feces. Walker-Smith wrote this to me after seeing this child initially in the outpatient clinic:

> *...there is a clear history of this child having been perfectly well until the age of 14 months and then the 2nd day after the MMR injection there was a change in behavior which has persisted thereafter and he has been diagnosed of having behavioral problems of autistic nature.*

Child 3's local pediatric neurologist, who was later to act as an expert on behalf of the vaccine manufacturers in the MMR litigation, was of a different opinion. He wrote:

> [Child 3's mother] *is devastated at the change in* [Child 3] *that occurred at around 14 months of age. She says this coincided with MMR immunization which she therefore blames... she is very sad and is looking both for somebody or something to blame and also for specific treatments for* [Child 3].

In further correspondence he wrote, with authority but, in my opinion, without appropriate investigation:

> *I have told them* [Child 3's parents] *that* [Child 3's] *acquired autistic problems in my opinion have occurred quite incidentally to his MMR immunisation rather than that they have been caused by this procedure.*

In her referral letter to Walker-Smith, Child 3's general practitioner (GP) was not so dismissive:

> [Child 3] *developed behavioural problems of autistic nature, severe constipation and learning difficulties after MMR vaccination. The batch incriminated was D1433, incidentally, which was the discontinued batch following adverse reactions.*

Child 3 was discharged from the Royal Free after only one follow-up visit due to the financial constraints imposed by his referring health authority. Walker-Smith wrote to the GP stating:

> *Our final diagnosis is of indeterminate ileocolitis*[5] *with lymphoid nodular hyperplasia*

Sadly, this child's neurologist was as dismissive of the expert interpretation of the intestinal findings as he had been of the mother's original story; he later declined to provide a prescription for Child 3's anti-inflammatory medication, writing:

> ...*clearly what Mrs.* [3] *wanted was a re-prescription for Salazopyrin*[6] *...this I am afraid I am not prepared to do... my difficulty is... the conceptual one of not accepting the concept of autistic enterocolitis.*[7]

Plans were put in place to follow up Child 3 locally in his hometown, but this proved unsatisfactory due to lack of adequate services. His continuing story reflects the tragedy of many of these children. His own particular *cri de coeur* – his attempt to communicate his pain and distress to others, which had started with his head-banging as an infant, further progressed by the time he was placed at the age of 12 into permanent care:

> [Child 3's] *behavior is extremely challenging by any standard... his behavior includes public masturbation, putting his finger up his anus and attempting to lick his fingers, spitting directly at people, biting his lip and spitting blood, hitting children and staff, forming a clenched fist and hitting, targeting women's breasts by hitting and pinching, kicking people and objects as he passes by, always throwing food or drink at people once he has sampled it, self-injurious hitting of upper arms and big toe, urinating on the carpet and furniture, smearing urine and feces on his body, breaking and tearing all objects including 1 TV, 4 cassette players, 2 windows, and 1 wall unit.* [Child 3's] *behavior is incessant...*

We will never know how much of this behavior had its roots in chronic physical pain and the failure of those around him to recognize this and act upon it. My experience of several thousand similarly affected children has persuaded me that a great deal of the behavioral component of this disorder is a response to pain – intestinal pain in particular. Time and again, I have seen these behaviors abate when the bowel disease has been treated.

As stated in Chapter 1 ("That Paper"), Child 4 has a particularly interesting and informative history. As a baby, it was noted that he had an unusually wide bridging of his nose. He was, therefore, followed closely for possible evidence of a congenital disorder, but this was excluded and he was discharged from follow-up as developmentally and physically normal by 15 months of age. He later received a single measles vaccine, following which he stopped cruising around furniture and regressed to crawling. He appeared to plateau in his learning, and by 20 months, he had lost the words that he had learned. Soon thereafter, he stopped talking altogether. General ill health developed in his second year with ear, chest, and throat infections and loose bowel motions with abdominal pain. According to his mother's story, 2 weeks following an MMR vaccine, at 4½ years of age, he "disappeared" and "lost all skills and communication." Whereas at 10 months of age he was able to build a tower of bricks, his play skills declined to the point that, according to his mother, "now he [was] lost as to what to do with them." In addition, he became clumsy, started head-banging, and developed repetitive behaviors typical of autism. He lost his self-help skills such that, whereas before the MMR he could feed himself with a spoon, afterwards he could no longer even hold a cup.

Child 4's GP highlighted the difficulties in providing a diagnostic label to this group of children, particularly those showing progressive deterioration over time, when in seeking help from an expert at the local university hospital he wrote:

> [Child 4's mother] *feels that he achieved certain milestones in the first year or two which were then lost subsequently but certainly by the age of four it was clear that* [Child 4] *had severe development delay. No specific diagnosis has ever been reached although assessment by a psychiatrist has agreed that he has many autistic tendencies... has also had recurrent problems with diarrhoea and has on occasions had infections which have been difficult to treat.*

This diagnostic uncertainty is also reflected in his pediatrician's letter to the local doctor in the local department of Community Child Health. Here we see others proposing a possible childhood disintegrative disorder (CDD) diagnosis (for more about this see Chapter 9, "The Devil's in the Detail") when she wrote:

> *"...the history does suggest features to suggest a disintegrative psychosis and there are certainly some autistic features in his behavior."* Another pediatrician later wrote: *"As* [Child 4] *grew older, it became clear that he had autism... However, such a diagnosis is not made instantly in the early years and both health professionals and parents seek alternative explanations. Also* [Child 4] *had a variety of rashes, abdominal pains and diarrhoea..."*

In fact, the diagnosis of autism was not made because, by virtue of the progressive and unusual nature of his deterioration, alternative "medical" explanations were more likely. Despite the clear clues, it does not seem that the search for alternative explanations was adequate. The history of Child 4's intestinal problems was also instructive. His records stated:

> The diarrhoea became a problem at between 1-1½ years of age [in fact, after his single measles vaccine]... it generally contains undigested food. His diarrhoea became significantly worse from 4½ years of age [after his MMR]...

Failure to thrive, a cardinal sign of pediatric inflammatory bowel disease, was evident from the family doctor's records where he was reported to be "dropping off centile charts." This failure to thrive continued and took another downturn at the same time his diarrhea worsened, when he was noted to have dropped from the 9th to the 2nd centile for weight.

Child 4 is particularly significant since he represents a possible *rechallenge* case. Rechallenge is the term used to describe a situation in which symptoms develop after an exposure, and after re-exposure to either the same or a similar factor (e.g., a measles-containing vaccine), there is an obvious recurrence or worsening of those symptoms. This specific set of circumstances is considered by the US Institute of Medicine to be powerful evidence of causation[8] and cannot be dismissed as coincidence. Despite this worrying sequence of events and the progressive deterioration of this little boy, none of this appeared to be of the least concern to anyone other than his parents and some of the doctors at the Royal Free.

Child 5's father made contact with me after reading a newspaper article about my work. His son had developed normally until he was 18 month old. That was the age at which he was given an MMR vaccine. Within 2 months, he started making strange noises and lost normal speech. He lost interest in his surroundings and became socially unresponsive. From 2 years of age he developed chronic alternating constipation and diarrhea as well as failure to thrive. A contrast X-ray of his intestine at the Royal Free identified a narrowing of his terminal ileum (the last part of his small intestine), which failed to dilate during the extended period of the investigation. While the appearances were consistent with Crohn's disease, the X-ray findings provided some diagnostic difficulties. His colonoscopy, however, confirmed the presence of a chronic inflammation.

Child 6 and Child 7 are brothers. Child 6, the older brother, suffered onset of rash, fever, drowsiness, aggressive behavior, and convulsions within 2 weeks of the MMR vaccine, followed by developmental regression. In addition, having been previously potty-trained, he became incontinent and his coordination deteriorated.[9] At the same time, he began to have abdominal pain, bloating and passage of mucus (a sign of inflammation) and blood per rectum, with alternating constipation and diarrhea. His blood markers of inflammation were raised,[10] and a colonoscopy revealed a marked colitis. Because of her concerns about the MMR vaccine and what appeared to have happened to her older son following vaccination, the mother of Child 7 decided not to give her younger son the MMR until he was 21 months old. She was finally persuaded that she was an irresponsible parent who was putting her infant boy at risk by not having him vaccinated. Tormented by guilt and still trusting of doctors over her own instincts, she took him for the vaccine. Within 1 month, he had become uncoordinated and had started losing skills. Like his brother, he had chronic unexplained alternating constipation and diarrhea with associated passage of blood and mucus. His blood tests revealed that he was anemic, and his inflammatory markers were raised.[11] Notably, however, his colonoscopy showed no evidence of inflammation, and the only finding at this stage was marked LNH of the ileum. His gastrointestinal symptoms worsened over the years and, unable to get the necessary investigations done in the UK, Mrs. 7 flew him to Austin, Texas, where he was reinvestigated at Thoughtful House Center for Children. He had a colonoscopy, and his biopsies were examined at an independent pathology laboratory. This time it was found that he had chronic active inflammation in his colon and stomach. It is possible but unlikely that this had been missed when he had his first colonoscopy at the Royal Free. What is more likely, in the light of experience, is that either in 1996 bowel inflammation was somewhere other than his colon or that in some children the disease progresses over time, potentially evolving on occasions into full-blown Crohn's disease.

Child 8's history required particularly careful attention. In her first year of life, Child 8's mother became concerned that she was not developing as rapidly as had her older sister. When she was 10 months old, she was referred to a developmental pediatrician. His expert opinion was that her developmental trajectory was normal. She was later diagnosed with coarctation of the aorta (a narrowing of the main artery leading from the heart). This was corrected by major surgery and she made an excellent recovery. From this point on, she made rapid gains in speech and other aspects of her development. Contemporaneous records described her mother as having been "delighted" with her subsequent progress. She received her MMR at the age of 18 months. Twenty-four hours later, she developed a rash and fever and started having febrile convulsions, requiring hospitalization for 5 days. Her regression followed immediately with behavioral deterioration, loss of words and vocalization, screaming, hyperacusis (an excessive sensitivity to sounds), loss of coordination[3] and nocturnal muscle jerks. There are multiple references in her medical records of her mother's clear association between her daughter's MMR vaccine and her dramatic deterioration. Interestingly, her GP had referred her for developmental follow-up at 17 months of age, just 1 month before her vaccine. The developmental pediatrician had assessed her and concluded that she was still developing normally, albeit at the slower end of the range, which was unsurprising in view of her aortic coarctation and major surgery. What is striking is that when she was reviewed again by the same developmental pediatrician a matter of weeks after her MMR vaccine, he considered her to be

> ...globally developmentally delayed functioning at about the one year level.

So it was that within the space of 1 month, Child 8 had gone from functioning at around the 17-month level down to the 12-month level, yet very little, if any, attention seems to have been paid to this. What is perhaps more surprising is that Professor Sir Michael Rutter, emeritus professor of child psychiatry and expert prosecution witness at the GMC, never having seen the child, felt able to offer the opinion that her regression was

> ...from a very low level.[12]

This was despite the fact that Child 8's developmental pediatrician had declared her slow but developmentally normal at 17 months of age. Child 8's reaction to the MMR was acknowledged but received no further consideration and no appropriate investigation until she arrived at the Royal Free. Her gastrointestinal symptoms followed a pattern that was, by now, becoming familiar, with the onset of chronic diarrhea. Her pediatric cardiologist noted mom's concern that

> ...she writhes and rolls around in her cot. Her mother wonders if something was "paining her."

And an entry in the GP's records documented the following:

> *...screaming constantly. Mum at end of tether...*

Her medical records contain numerous additional references to Child 8's continuing gastrointestinal issues, about which there was otherwise precious little professional interest until she made contact with the Royal Free.

Child 8 was assessed by a child psychiatrist at the Royal Free who was candid about the likely role of MMR in this child's regression:

> *...I note that following the vaccination there was a period of fever, diarrhoea and developmental regression. I am therefore left wondering whether in fact she had post vaccination encephalitis...*

At that time, he did not consider her to be autistic, although she was later diagnosed independently with autism at another university hospital. Despite a documented loss of 5 months of development in just 1 month, Rutter was unimpressed by Child 8's developmental course, as captured in his report:[13]

> *The slight regression following MMR was, understandably, a cause for concern for the parents but was **not of a form or degree that carried much clinical meaning.**[14]*

As the MMR issue later reached a political fever pitch, there was an exchange of correspondence between Child 8's GP and her developmental pediatrician who wrote, in a state of almost tangible agitation:

> *...On reviewing her records I find that the concern about [Child 8's] developmental delay was expressed by her mother and yourself in May 1994, long before the MMR was given in January or February 1995. The fever-associated convulsion which she had in February 1995 was in the context of a diarrhoeal illness associated with fever two weeks after her MMR immunisation. I feel therefore that it is extremely unlikely that the MMR was the cause of her present problems...*

This pediatrician appears to have ignored his own assessments of Child 8 that showed clear deterioration after the vaccine. The early concerns about Child 8's development were reported accurately in *The Lancet*. In spite of this, however, in her evidence to the GMC, Child 8's GP felt able, without having read the paper in detail (as she admitted), to voice her concern to the prosecution that we had reported this little girl's early development as "normal." We had not. Despite having no basis in fact, this effectively amounted to an allegation of scientific fraud.

Child 9's mother was friendly with Rosemary Kessick. His story is a further indictment of the medical profession. As it was originally told to us by his mother, Child 9's story was one of normal development followed by developmental regression from 18 months of age after one in a series of many episodes of middle ear infection. His regression, described by several doctors as "secondary autism"[15] consisted of a gradual deterioration with physical regression and loss of coordination – he could no longer throw and catch a ball, his gait became "awkward and stiff like an old man," and he could no longer go from sitting to standing unaided. He lost the 20 words that he had gained and developed secondary fecal incontinence. His play skills evaporated, leaving his older sister feeling confused and rejected. He began to have episodes of severe abdominal pain associated with screaming and with bringing his knees up to his chest and rolling from one side of the bed to the other. From approximately 2 years of age, he developed a pattern of chronic loose bowel motions containing undigested food. He fell from the 97th centile for weight at 1 year old to the 50th by 2 years old. His diet went from being varied to very restricted, consisting of refined carbohydrates and at least ten 200 ml cartons of a synthetic orange-flavored drink per day.

During one particularly severe bout of abdominal pain, the family doctor was called. She attempted to examine Child 9's abdomen on the basis that this was evidently the source of his pain. Unable to, she examined his ears, declared one eardrum "pink" and prescribed a powerful broad-spectrum antibiotic for a presumed ear infection, ignoring the abdominal problem altogether. The GP continued in this way, prescribing antibiotics on a monthly basis, until Child 9's mother stopped consulting this doctor. She said:

> I stopped consulting her as her attitude as with many other doctors had become "he is autistic" his problem is behavioural not pain.

As explained previously in Chapter 1 ("That Paper"), what Child 9's mother did not tell us in 1996 was that she, too, had linked her son's problems contemporaneously to MMR vaccine. Our description of this child in *The Lancet* faithfully reiterated the onset of symptoms following an episode of otitis media and made no mention of the MMR. The reason for the discordance between these two aspects of the narrative provides a valuable lesson. When she had first approached her son's pediatrician with the possibility that his problems stemmed from MMR, he had been dismissive. Other doctors had reacted in the same way. When Child 9's parents took their son to be assessed by a developmental pediatrician at a university hospital, he said with certainty,

> My dear, I have sat on the Vaccine Damage Board for several years and vaccines do not cause autism.

He did offer the family an alternative: if they looked back into their family histories, then they would probably find at least one family member who had similar symptoms. Diligently, they did so. Child 9's mother was one of eight children and both of her parents were one of ten children. Her maternal grandfather was one of fifteen boys. Her husband's paternal grandmother was one of twenty-one children. In spite of such enthusiastic procreation, neither autism nor anything resembling it had ever been an issue on either side of the family. Nonetheless, beyond that point, Child 9's father urged his wife not to mention the MMR again since doctors considered her to be crazy.

Here was a situation where the mother's original narrative – that which should have been key to understanding the origin of her son's problems – had been dismissed or scorned, causing her to modify her story (quite understandably, but to Medicine's enduring shame) in order not to compromise her son's access to clinical care.

Child 10 received his MMR at 12 months of age and developed entirely normally for a further 4 months. After an apparent measles infection at 16 months of age, he developed a rash, fever, vomiting, and reduced level of consciousness. Over the following 4 months he progressively lost eye contact, verbal skills, interest in play and socialization, and developed repetitive behaviors. A consultant pediatric neurologist wrote:

> It seems that [Child 10's] strange behaviour started after he had an illness which was considered likely to have been measles and which occurred in June 1994.

As was commonplace in the diagnostic maze of child psychiatry, on separate occasions he was diagnosed variously with autism, disintegrative disorder, and encephalitis leading to generalized brain disorder. Once again, in parallel with his developmental regression he developed abdominal pain, diarrhea, and intolerance for certain foods.

Despite the fact that no definitive tests had been performed at the time of his possible measles infection at 16 months, a strong indication that this diagnosis was, in fact, correct was his hugely elevated measles antibody level. Levels such as those in Child 10 (that have remained high for many years) are only seen in a rare form of measles encephalitis,[16] although there has been no further indication that this is what he has. If correct, then his physical and immunological reaction may have occurred following natural exposure at 16 months due to a primary vaccine failure (i.e., his MMR did not protect him), or his measles infection at 16 months was, in fact, a reactivation of vaccine virus infection.

In assessing Child 10 at the Royal Free, our child psychiatrist documented:

> *He is far too affectionate by his father's account for a child with full blown autism… I thought the most likely diagnosis was in fact an encephalitic episode, which led to some low grade generalized brain damage.*

Despite this, he subsequently received an autism diagnosis from several other experts. For the Royal Free child psychiatrist, the demonstration of affection appeared to be a sticking point. In psychiatrist and physician Leo Kanner's original description of autism in 1943 and in much of the literature thereafter, children with autism are characterized as aloof and relatively undemonstrative. This may be the case when their autism has followed an exposure in the womb or in perinatal life when there has been no opportunity to bond or experience the shared rewards of affection. If, however, a child's emotions have developed normally for 16 months, then while other aspects of cognition may regress and behaviors change, it is quite possible that affection — by this stage firmly entrenched — still remains.

Austrian educator Theodore Heller's original description in 1908 reveals that children with CDD may be capable of expressing affection.[17] A 1996 paper from Russo and colleagues that detailed a case of CDD and provided a review of the medical literature on this disease discusses the presentation of the condition and the close overlap with the symptoms of autism. The key features they describe in the child's history included normal early development, progressive loss of speech and language, development of restricted interests, repetitive behaviors, secondary urinary and fecal incontinence, spontaneous inconsolable crying episodes, and loss of self-help skills. Despite this, he remained affectionate and was happy between crying episodes.

In addition to Child 10's displays of affection, his presentation was very much like that of Russo's case, and this was characterized in correspondence from his local consultant community pediatrician. He wrote:

> [Child 10's GP] *asked me to see* [him] *urgently because of concerns about his development going backwards and because he seems to have lost some speech and social skills... he was a perfectly normal healthy lad until June 1994... following his episode of measles* [Child 10] *appeared to lose eye contact, he fell into his own world, lost interest in his toys and books, and ceased almost all interaction with other people. His early vocalizations ceased, his mother wasn't sure if he was deaf or simply not understanding... developed a habit of bouncing up and down, jiggling, clinging, and running in circles and banging and kicking in the cot for an hour or so... it is interesting that he has intermittent episodes of watery diarrhea and has episodes of screaming when he clutches his abdomen which could be related to abdominal pain.*

There was little, if anything, that distinguished this child from the others seen at the Royal Free. While the onset of CDD after measles is recognized in the medical literature, the little known fact that onset after immunization has also been described quite independently of the Royal Free will not surprise the parents of affected children.[18]

Child 10 likewise turned out to have a low-grade colitis and LNH. On the anti-inflammatory Salazopyrin, his diarrhea and pain were reported in his chart to be "much improved."

Child 11 was our first referral from the US. He came to us with a history of developmental regression starting at 18 months of age; this included loss of speech, repetitive hand movements, and reduced eye contact and progressed to complete loss of speech by 30 months of age. At 3 years old he was described as having the cognitive function of a 6-month-old. He was particularly intolerant of certain foods, with worsening of behaviors in response to bread, dairy products, and confectionary. His findings at colonoscopy of LNH and a low-grade colitis were consistent with the emerging pattern seen in other, similarly affected children.

Child 12's mother met the mother of Child 6 and Child 7 at a playgroup for special needs children. They talked about their children and, in particular, the latter mother's experience at the Royal Free. Child 12's mother subsequently made contact with me by telephone. Her son had developed normally to just over 16 months of age when he had a series of nonspecific illnesses suggestive of viral infection. This had been detailed as part of the South Thames Development & Communication Study being undertaken at Guy's Hospital in London, where he was given his developmental diagnosis. He had received his MMR vaccine at 15 months of age, but his mother did not link this to his subsequent regression. However, his GP noted this in Child 12's medical records:

...frequent illnesses since MMR.

Child 12 also developed a measles-like disease at 20 months of age, although no attempt to confirm or refute this was made. Susceptibility to recurrent infections was a feature of many affected children and reinforced the impression of a fundamental problem with their immune systems. Child 12's developmental diagnosis was Asperger's syndrome,[19] a condition on the autism continuum that is often referred to as being at the high-functioning end of the spectrum. A fundamental aspect of Asperger's that distinguishes it from autism is the normal acquisition of speech, and a diagnosis of Asperger's requires cognitive function within the normal range for age.

It would be a mistake to consider Asperger's syndrome to be a mild form of autism. Dr. Marcel Kinsbourne, a pediatric neurologist and someone who has done more to support the cause of vaccine-damaged children than anyone else, pointed this error out to me. Asperger's sufferers attend regular school, where they may well excel academically. However, mainstream school can be a brutal environment for those who are socially isolated, lack empathy, and miss the cues and clues that designate one as "cool." To wear a virtual badge that says "odd" in the teenage years, in particular — and to know it — is a heavy cross to bear.

Child 12's developmental regression started with loss of speech, decreased social awareness and interaction, and deteriorating coordination at 16 months of age. At the same time, he suffered onset of unexplained chronic abdominal pain, constipation, secondary fecal incontinence, vomiting, and loss of appetite. His bowel movements were pale, loose, and very offensive, which are characteristic features of malabsorption. Consistent with a diagnosis of malabsorption was his failure, according to his chart, "to grow or put on weight." Blood markers, measured before and after his admission to the Royal Free, showed evidence of inflammation. His biopsies showed a mild colitis, and he responded well to anti-inflammatory medication.

So, what were we to make of these stories? From modern medicine's classical roots, pattern recognition has been a fundamental part of good medical practice and essential in the detection and description of new disease syndromes. Emergent patterns will have been evident to those reading the children's stories above. Genius is not required, but skilled, unbiased attention to the history and clinical findings is. Unlike family doctors, who may only have seen one or two autistic children in their practice by the mid-'90s, from July 1996, we, in a tertiary referral center, had the advantage of a repetitious and intensive exposure to the myriad problems from which these children suffered. As such, it was our duty as well as readily within our grasp to recognize and document emergent patterns of disease presentation.

Patterns also emerge in, for example, blood tests, which when viewed as a whole are more meaningful than when observed in isolation. Iron deficiency of a mild but consistent degree was present in many children, indicative of either low dietary iron intake, malabsorption from a diseased intestine, or blood loss. Vitamin B12 levels were, in fact, high in the blood plasma of these children. Other than in the case of Child 9, the problem did not appear to be one of impaired B12 absorption from the intestine but a more subtle abnormality of B12 metabolism in the body's cells. The B12 in the children's blood, although high, was in a useless, inactive form and was raised because, when not complexed[20] inside the cells, it leaks out of the cells into the blood plasma. Dr. John Linnell, a biochemist on the team, identified an abnormally high level of the vitamin B12 metabolite methylmalonic acid (MMA) in the children's urine. The raised MMA level reflected an abnormal B12 metabolism. What is fascinating is that this fact, unearthed by the Royal Free team back in the late 1990s, has now captured the interest of many in the autism scientific and medical communities; this has led to therapeutic trials of the active form of B12 that are underway in hopes of overcoming this problem.

There are also those idiosyncratic features of the children's behavior that turned out to be related to gastrointestinal distress. They included posturing, a behavior that often involved leaning for hours at a time over the edge of a piece of furniture that was, as it turned out, done in order to apply pressure to the abdomen and relieve their pain. Such behaviors continue to be misinterpreted as "Oh, that's just his autism," when, in fact, they are entirely appropriate for a child with abdominal pain who can find no other form of expression or relief. Many children became particularly agitated when they needed to go to the toilet, when characteristic features of autism such as hand flapping would intensify.

Other behaviors included food refusal or selectivity, with a particular preference for large volumes of cow's milk and refined carbohydrates, and extreme thirst. Paradoxically, the past medical history often involved intolerance of cow's milk in infancy, with reflux[21] (heartburn) and projectile vomiting. Sleep disturbances, often associated with reflux, were very common, illustrated by children who had previously slept through the night falling into a pattern of waking frequently in distress.

Most interesting mechanistically was the aberrant or aggravated behavioral response to certain foods and, as a logical extension to this, the beneficial effect of excluding these foods from the child's diet. Gluten, a protein derived from cereals, and casein from cow's milk, seemed two of the most frequently cited culprits. Whatever the mechanism or mechanisms, we were rapidly persuaded by video and other evidence that the effect of withdrawing these substrates from the diet could lead to benefit. Following inadvertent reintroduction of these foodstuffs, the subsequent deterioration in symptoms – a rechallenge phenomenon – has convinced me further of their biological effect in many affected children.

Multiple courses of antibiotics, given routinely as a panacea for presumed middle ear infections, were also a recurring feature. This, combined with a frequent history of eczema, hay fever, and surgery to remove tonsils and adenoids, suggested strongly that there was an underlying immunological vulnerability in many of these children.

Also striking were parental reports of cognitive improvement and even "normalization" during periods of high fever. The story was far too common and consistent among disparate groups of parents to be simply a chance occurrence. This change in behavior with fever has since been documented in the medical literature by autism researchers at Kennedy Krieger Institute and Johns Hopkins in Baltimore.[22] It provides a crucial clue as to the reversibility of aspects of a disease previously deemed irreversible by many "experts."

Changes in sensory perception were also issues that I had not encountered in the medical textbooks. On a hot day, the child would be wrapped in three layers of clothes, and yet on a freezing cold day, they would be running around naked in the snow. Changes in a child's perception of pain were common, with an extremely high threshold in many cases. A child might burn themselves on an electric ring or a boiling kettle and yet barely acknowledge the fact. There is no easy explanation for such changes although many more or less plausible mechanisms have been posited.

Turning to the vexed subject of MMR vaccine, certain consistent features emerged over the years that, while difficult to interpret in the absence of a non-autistic comparison group, certainly raised questions about a cause-effect relationship. Affected children had often been vaccinated while unwell with fever or while on antibiotics. Some had mistakenly received two doses of the vaccine in quick succession or were given many vaccines, including MMR, on the same day – in the absence of any safety studies – merely for the sake of convenience. Many of the more severely affected children were rechallenge cases who, despite regression following the first dose, had been given a booster MMR with catastrophic consequences. I was later to discover, to my dismay, that this applied to Child 2. In combing through his records, I found a signed consent form for an MMR vaccination when he was only 4 months of age. Given the knowledge that risks from many viruses such as measles are greatest in the very young, this vaccination strategy borders on insanity. My suspicions are that he was part of an experimental trial that went badly wrong and has never been reported. I suspect this because at that time, another mother from the same part of the country as Child 2 was invited to have her own son participate in an experimental trial of MMR vaccine in infants. Apparently, this vaccine trial was abandoned, and when one of the nurses involved in the trial offered to disclose the details to this mother, she was threatened with loss of her job.

Clumsiness was a significant symptom in several respects, firstly because it confirmed an encephalopathy – brain dysfunction – in these children that went way beyond behavioral aberrations. Secondly, a particular form of clumsiness, *cerebellar ataxia* (incoordination originating due to malfunctioning of a part of the brain called the cerebellum), has been described as a complication of MMR vaccination. This pattern of clumsiness was consistent with the problems suffered by these children. Cerebellar ataxia was first reported as a possible complication of MMR by Dr. Anne-Marie Plesner in Denmark.[23] This association had not been detected with any other vaccine administered to children of the same age, including the single measles vaccine, indicating that a novel adverse reaction might be associated with the combined MMR vaccine. In a more recent follow-up of the mandatory passive reporting system operated in Denmark, Plesner not only confirmed this association, but also indicated that the more severe ataxias following MMR were associated with residual cognitive deficits in some children.[24] This sounds suspiciously like our own experience.

Then there are those completely unexpected symptom patterns that emerge by virtue of one's investigation and treatment that, while not anticipated, provide an exquisite insight into, for example, the relationship between bowel, brain, and behavior. When the children were first admitted to the Royal Free as outpatients, we anticipated mayhem on the wards. Colonoscopy requires a bowel prep that clears out the colon and allows the entire length of the large intestine to be visualized. Although children usually tolerate this preparation very well, we had anticipated problems and a big cleaning bill from giving powerful laxatives to non-potty-trained children who were in a state of perpetual motion. To our surprise, however, parents reported that their child had never been calmer and their stay in hospital with their child was like a holiday. Resting the bowel by not eating for 24 hours combined with bowel clearance of substances that were potentially inflammatory or toxic might explain this phenomenon. It certainly reinforced to us the reality of a gut-brain interaction in this disease. The same beneficial effect on both bowel and behavioral symptoms was seen with anti-inflammatory medication used to treat the intestinal inflammation. This benefit was very common — although not universal, and when it occurred, it seemed to go beyond the simple relief of pain. We tried for years to examine this effect in a controlled clinical trial, but by this time and for various reasons, funding was becoming more and more difficult to come by.

The thing about pattern recognition is that, for the process to be enabled, one has to *allow* the line of enquiry; that is, one has to explore a symptom or pursue an aspect of the past medical history through the narrative maze to a final, considered determination of its significance. There are several constraints on this process, none of which make for good medicine. The first is the view that the "doctor knows best," even for a disease like autism about which so much remains to be discovered. The doctor seems deaf, even hostile, to anything outside his or her specific realm of interest or belief system. The second constraint is the sheer, unmitigated fear of calling MMR vaccine safety into question.

So, where are these children now? I am sad to say that despite our best efforts and some early symptomatic improvement, the prognosis for at least the majority of these children remains very guarded. Some have been institutionalized, and for the rest of them, this is a possibility unless something dramatic changes. Whatever happens, none will function and be safe independently outside of long-term supervision in a protected environment. At least four have developed epilepsy. For others, like Child 7, the bowel disease appears to have progressed. Who knows how they would be now had they not been treated? Their prognosis was – and remains – an unknown quantity, particularly since we do not know the natural history of the intestinal inflammation. The issue of prognosis was raised when our application to the ethics committee was first reviewed and was one that was to resurface in the GMC hearing in the guise of alleged professional misconduct.

Back in 1996, in response to a question from a lay member of the Royal Free Hospital's ethics committee about whether an intensive regime of investigation was justified, Walker-Smith replied, with the sincerity of a man who has devoted his professional life to the care of sick children:

> These children suffer from a disease with a "hopeless prognosis" in relation to their cerebral disintegrative disorder. They have often not had the level of investigation which we would regard as adequate for a child presenting with such a devastating condition.

He was generous in his restraint when stating:

> In relation to their gastrointestinal symptoms, which will be present in all the children we investigate, these have often been under-investigated.

The integrity and compassion that underpinned his position should have been unassailable. Nonetheless, at the GMC hearing many years later, the prosecution accused Walker-Smith of having sought to mislead the ethics committee in order to advance "experimentation" on these children by misrepresenting their long-term outcome. Unrestrainedly cynical, the prosecuting counsel, Sallie Smith, QC, painted a picture of the exploitation of desperate children, labeled falsely by Walker-Smith with a "hopeless prognosis." Smith was supported in her case by Rutter, despite the fact that by his own admission, none of the children had shown any signs of lasting neurological recovery. Indeed, many had deteriorated further from an already severe state.

Walker-Smith was right; without help – help in the broadest sense of painstaking medical enquiry and multiple levels of intervention – "hopeless" anticipated a lifetime of isolation, incarceration, and pain. In his response to the ethics committee, Walker-Smith captured, with vivid clarity, these children's futures.

Nonetheless, there is hope, and this is growing as the medical community wakes up to its responsibilities. The legacy of the children in the vanguard of these discoveries is a better chance for those who have followed them. I have hope, not least because I have come to believe that the disease is deceptive: it creates the illusion of a brain injury that appears more pervasive and intractable than it really is. Sometimes, if we care to, we can accept an insight offered in the moment, as important as it is evanescent. Once, at the house of a friend in Sacramento, California, we were by the pool in the late afternoon when he asked his profoundly autistic son if he wanted to go to a popular restaurant for dinner. The boy stopped dead in his tracks; his persistent repetitive hand movements ceased; and he focused — tangibly focused – on finding a way of getting his answer out. He had understood the question and he wanted to take his father up on the offer, but he had no way of telling him. The wiring that linked his hearing and understanding of the question to the brain centers responsible for articulating and vocalizing his answer was shorting out at some point. Eventually, he took his father by the hand and led him to the car; he had found a way. And we, too, must find a way.

Postscript
At the GMC, my response to the parents' pleas for help – a recommendation that they seek referral to Walker-Smith and my offer to provide some explanation to their family doctor by way of collegial communication – was somehow twisted and repackaged to appear as a cynical misdemeanor. What was no more than a professional and humane response to a cry from the heart became part of a grand conspiracy to "cherry-pick" children for the purpose of experimentation.

The alternative course to me, having listened to the parents of *The Lancet 12* and many more besides, and having acknowledged their desperate plight, the various violations of their children's rights, the willful ignorance that often confronted their insights and suspicions, and their tears – would have been to tell them to go away and not to bother me any further. Ironically, this behavior, while it might smack of "callous disregard" would, it appears, have been preferable to the GMC and would not have brought me to its doors.

Endnotes

[1] Magnetic resonance imaging of the brain.

[2] Electroencephalogram: electrical recording of the brain.

[3] Seen by Dr. John Hunter who writes to JWS. ESR 40.

[4] Walker-Smith JA, et al. Ileo-caecal lymphoid nodular hyperplasia non-specific ileo-colitis with regressive behavioural disorder and food intolerance: A case study. *J Pediatr Gastroenterol Nutr.* 1997;25(Suppl 1): S48.

[5] Inflammation of the small and large intestine.

[6] AKA sulfasalazine.

[7] Autistic enterocolitis is the name given to the pattern of bowel inflammation in children with autism.

[8] Stratton K et al. *Adverse Events Associated with Childhood Vaccines: Evidence Bearing on Causality.* Washington, D.C.: National Academy Press,1994.

[9] For further information on ataxia following MMR vaccination see: Plesner AM. Gait disturbance after measles mumps rubella vaccine. *Lancet* 1995;345:316. This was later confirmed in follow-up study: Plesner AM, Hansen FJ, Taadon K, et al. Gait disturbance interpreted as cerebellar ataxia after MMR vaccination at 15 months of age: a follow-up study. *Acta Paediatrica.* 2000;89:58-63.

[10] Raised ESR (31); raised platelet count (480).

[11] January 28, 1997 (scope January 26, 1997): Hemoglobin 10.6/9.4 [1.97 on ward] (persistent microcytic anaemia); WBC 17.2, ESR 16. platelets 340, barium meal and FT (29.1.97. LNH).

[12] Rutter report to Field Fisher Waterhouse. May 7, 2007. Page 4.

[13] Rutter report to Field Fisher Waterhouse. May 7, 2007. Page 5.

[14] Emphasis added.

[15] Autism occurring in a previously developmentally normal child.

[16] Subacute sclerosing panencephalitis.

[17] Heller T. Dementia infantilis, *Zeitschrift fur die Erforschung und Behandlung des Jugen lichen Schwansinns.* 1908;2:141-165.

[18] In a report of 12 cases in India seen between 1989 and 1998, Malhotra and Gupta note onset in 4 cases following infectious/vaccine exposures, including fever with seizures, acute gastroenteritis and vaccination. The type of vaccine is not stated. See: Malhotra S and Gupta N. Childhood disintegrative disorder. Re-examination of the current concept. *Eur J Child and Adolescent Psych.* 2002;11:108-114.

[19] Asperger published the first definition of Asperger syndrome in 1944. In four boys, he identified a pattern of behavior and abilities that he called "autistic psychopathy," meaning autism (self) and psychopathy (personality disease). The pattern included

"a lack of empathy, little ability to form friendships, one-sided conversation, intense absorption in a special interest, and clumsy movements."

The term "Asperger's syndrome" was popularized in a 1981 paper by British researcher Lorna Wing, which challenged the previously accepted model of autism presented by Leo Kanner in 1943. Unlike Kanner, Hans Asperger's findings were ignored and disregarded in the English-speaking world in his lifetime. See also: Asperger H.[On the differential diagnosis of early infantile autism] (in German). *Acta Paedopsychiatr.* 1968;35(4): 136–45.

[20] As methylcobalamin.

[21] Gastroesophageal reflux involves an abnormal backward flow of gastric juices (acid) into the esophagus, causing inflammation and pain. This is particularly likely to occur at night causing waking and distress.

[22] Curran LK. et al. Behaviors Associated with Fever in Children with Autism Spectrum Disorders. *Pediatrics.* 2007:120(6);e1386-e1392.

[23] Plesner AM. Gait disturbance after measles mumps rubella vaccine. *The Lancet* 1995;345:316, and Plesner AM, Hansen FJ, Taadon K, Nielson LH, Larsen CB, Pedersen E. Gait disturbance interpreted as cerebellar ataxia after MMR vaccination at 15 months of age: a follow-up study. *Acta Paediatrica.* 2000;89:58-63.

[24] Plesner AM, Hansen FJ, Taadon K, Nielson LH, Larsen CB, Pedersen E. Gait disturbance interpreted as cerebellar ataxia after MMR vaccination at 15 months of age: a follow-up study. *Acta Paediatrica.* 2000;89:58-63.

CHAPTER THREE

The Dean's Dilemma

And then there was the spawning of what was rapidly to become a ruthlessly pragmatic effort to put an end to my group's vaccine safety research. There were at least two shades of irony that played out in the unfolding drama. One was behind the scenes, the covert action that was unknown to me at the time. The other involved the mechanism by which this covert action was revealed – none of it would ever have come to light were it not for the allegations made by the freelance journalist Brian Deer and his complaints to the GMC. The disclosures included documents – thousands of them – that some must have hoped would never surface. But surface they did, like bloated corpses from the river bed. The evidence revealed collusion at the highest levels of the medical establishment (see below and Chapter 6, "The Dean's Press Briefing").

During the first half of 1996, I was asked for help by Richard Barr of Dawbarn's law firm and lead attorney on the UK MMR cases. Specifically, I was asked to review the safety of measles-containing vaccines (MCV) and, separately, to design a study that would help determine whether there was or was not a likely case in law against the manufacturers of MCV. Barr's initial interest was in Crohn's disease as a possible adverse outcome, but autism in children with intestinal symptoms rapidly took center stage. I prepared a research proposal for Barr's submission to the Legal Aid Board (LAB), a means-tested, government-funded legal assistance program to which Barr was contracted for the vaccine work. The proposal focused upon laboratory-based detection of measles virus in the diseased intestinal tissues of children with Crohn's disease and those with developmental disorder and intestinal symptoms, should they come to colonoscopy. I anticipated that the laboratory work would take 1 year; in the event, it required 2 years.

When confirmation of the award of the LAB research grant came from Barr in August 1996, I was out of the country. Upon my return, I wrote to a Dave Wilson in the finance department of the Royal Free Hospital School of Medicine on September 26 to say,

...we have recently been awarded a grant from the Legal Aid Board to fund research into measles virus and IBD.

So, no secret there.[1] I attached the letter of award that the LAB had written to the law firm, Dawbarns, and confirmed that the first £25,000.00 should be paid into a designated research account as was standard practice for research grants. On the same day, I wrote to Barr asking if the funds could be transferred to the medical school.

But in September 1996, what I did not know was that to Professor Arie Zuckerman, the dean of the medical school, my agreement to act on behalf of vaccine-damaged children was old news. In fact, he had known about it for some months, having been informed by Professor Sir David Hull, the then-chairman of the Joint Committee on Vaccination and Immunisation (JCVI) and another person at the UK's Department of Heath (DoH).[2] It appears the DoH was eager for Zuckerman to know of my intentions and wanted him to bring to bear whatever pressure he could in order to stop me.

In early March 1997, I received a call from Zuckerman. The details of this conversation can be gleaned from our subsequent correspondence on the matter. In a letter dated March 10, 1997, I sought to respond to the matters that he had raised. He was under the impression that there was a parliamentary select committee (the equivalent of an oversight committee hearing) being convened to address the subject of measles vaccine and Crohn's disease and, seemingly, my link with the solicitors, Dawbarns. I will set out verbatim the remainder of my response here:

> *You mentioned a conflict of interest when we spoke. This is something which has exercised my mind greatly in the interim. I feel I must go on record as stating that I do not see how any conflict of interest exists. It is, as I am sure you would agree, our joint and several responsibilities as members of the medical profession to use our training and expertise appropriately. In the context of the current measles vaccine safety/ consequences debate, I am providing independent expert guidance based on facts available to me. I do this in common with colleagues worldwide...*

> *...In the particular circumstances with which I am dealing, there is, I believe, an even higher moral obligation to act as an expert adviser. We are faced with a situation where the most vulnerable category of patients, i.e. children, may be put at risk. It is right and proper therefore to review the facts, assess them, and offer guidance.*

I hope these comments are helpful. Please do feel free to contact me if you wish to discuss my role further.

In our telephone exchange, Zuckerman appeared tormented by the issue of conflict of interest but failed to specify what this conflict might be. In his response of March 13, he denied there ever having been a parliamentary select committee enquiry on this matter. He continued:

I do not think that there is any conflict between duty of care to patients or the provision of independent expert advice to lawyers. However, it is a different matter when lawyers fund a particular piece of research where a specific action is contemplated. This surely suggests that some preliminary legal discussions have taken place and that a specific action is contemplated. If so, then the interpretation must surely be that a conflict of interest may well exist. The School must, therefore, seek expert advice, but in the meantime you should know of my concern.[4]

At the time, I did not understand his rather convoluted reasoning. My inference was that he objected fundamentally to the funding of research by lawyers acting on behalf of children who might have been damaged by a vaccine.

Clinical trials of vaccines and drugs are funded by the manufacturers for the principal purpose of profit. This is not a judgment or a criticism, but an economic reality for an industry that is answerable first and foremost to its stockholders. It appeared to me that, unspoken, Zuckerman was proffering the ethical paradox of medical academia endorsing – indeed embracing – the conduct of clinical trials funded by the pharmaceutical industry, but denouncing as something distasteful and prohibitively conflicted[17] the investigation of children whose lives may have been irreparably damaged by an inadequately tested vaccine.

Let me deal with the specifics of his reasoning: "it is a different matter when lawyers fund a particular piece of research where a specific action is contemplated." In the context of a drug trial, the "piece of research," would be the drug trial, and when a "specific action is contemplated," this would constitute the potential for subsequent marketing of the drug. Let's move on to his words "This surely suggests that some preliminary legal discussions have taken place and that a specific action is contemplated." One can apply the same logic to a drug trial: preliminary discussions inevitably take place in the assessment of the trial's feasibility, once again, in the anticipation that if the trial goes ahead and is successful, a profitable drug will be brought to market.

The "conflict of interest" is properly dealt with in any presentation and publication of the study's results by disclosing the fact that the trial was funded by a pharmaceutical company. Was there anything other than profit versus compensation that separated these two seemingly concordant research strategies? What was actually troubling Zuckerman so profoundly? Perhaps I was missing something. Confused by his lack of clarity over this supposed conflict, I wrote again on March 24, 1997. I enclosed all the documents relevant to the grant, including the proposal, the letters from the LAB, and the relevant protocols – once again there was no secrecy in terms of frankly telling the dean what was proposed. In an effort to assuage his fears, I continued:

> *I got the impression from Roy* [Professor Pounder] *that you were concerned that we were being contracted to provide a specific answer – that is, that measles vaccine or the MMR vaccine was the cause of this disease. That is absolutely not the case. We are being funded to conduct a piece of scientific research to establish or refute the link between MMR vaccine and the disease. There are absolutely no preconditions concerning the outcome. If this were the case, you may rest assured I would have never been involved in the first instance. The science must lead and everything else follows. As with the medical expert's opinion elsewhere, I am being asked to provide my opinion, whether that opinion is positive or negative. It is on this basis, and only on this basis, that I have agreed to assist in this matter. I hope that his issue can be resolved as quickly as possible and my group is working to achieve this end.*

It was years later that I found out the reasoning behind Zuckerman's fears and why the DoH was so highly motivated to stop the vaccine safety research. That reason was most alarming – the DoH stood to be sued. For reasons unknown to me, Barr and his legal team, the LAB, and the parents who were contemplating legal redress for their children's injuries, it was not just big pharma but a department of Her Majesty's Government that was in the firing line.

But back in 1996 this information was not intended for me. None of us were intended to know then. None of us were *ever* intended to know. This is evident inasmuch as it was never spontaneously disclosed. So it was that, rather than raise any concerns about the LAB grant with me,

Zuckerman had been hard at work exploring possible grounds for refusing the funding, which would have then compromised this specific research, something that would have pleased his political friends. As his line of attack, he chose the ethical implications of the LAB funding a piece of medical research. On October 11, 1996, he wrote to Dr. Mac Armstrong, chairman of the ethics committee of the British Medical Association (BMA),[3] the UK's professional organization for doctors:

> *I should be grateful for your advice on a potentially difficult situation in which the Royal Free finds itself and on which therefore I must take a decision on the position adopted by the Medical School. A senior member of the School's clinical academic staff is engaged in work that has become somewhat controversial in that he is suggesting a causal link between the measles virus and in particular vaccination against measles and the onset of Crohn's disease and inflammatory bowel disorders. Arising from recent widespread publicity given to this research, the Legal Aid Board has provided funding through a firm of solicitors representing Crohn's disease sufferers and we have been asked to make an appointment to the staff of the Medical School specifically to undertake a pilot study of selected patients. **Clearly this could lead to a case against the Government for damages.**[7]*

Here Zuckerman's motive – preventing a case against the government – was revealed, but why this little known fact should have been clear to Armstrong at this stage is uncertain. In contrast with the US, where legal claims for possible vaccine damage are routinely filed against the government, this is not the case in the UK where the anticipated legal action was to have been against the vaccine manufacturer.

Zuckerman continued:

> *My dilemma is that the Medical School might be seen to utilise its resources which are largely funded from the public purse to take sides in litigation before there has been a finding. It is quite common of course for clinical academic staff to be called as expert witnesses in cases criminal and civil where they act as individuals although their reputation is clearly based in large measure upon their academic and professional appointments. This is however a somewhat different situation and I would find it helpful if you could let me know whether you have come across parallels elsewhere that might provide a precedent and also advise me on the ethical and legal position of the Medical School.*

Not surprisingly Armstrong was somewhat bemused and wrote to Zuckerman on October 15, 1996, to try and gain some further information upon which to base his advice.

While this was all going on behind the scenes, the check from the LAB, via Dawbarns, was sent to me on December 6, 1996. As outlined earlier, unaware of the machinations that had been set in place, I forwarded the check to Wilson in finance, reiterating the source and purpose of the funds. Wilson then copied this to the medical school secretary, Brian Blatch, on December 12 with a memo that read:

> Following on from our discussion yesterday I thought it prudent that you should have previous correspondence on the issues raised so far so that you are aware of the present state of play.

Clearly this source of funding had enlivened the finance department. Although working like a well-oiled machine when dealing with checks from the pharmaceutical industry, they were thrown into confusion by a research grant from the LAB. Annotations that were added to Wilson's memo in an anxious hand read:

> "We cannot code the cheque. We may have to return it." Beneath that, someone called Renee had written, "We have already banked check."

In fact, Zuckerman, while soliciting the expert advice of the BMA's ethics committee, had put a block on the research by placing the funds in an inaccessible *suspense* account. I knew nothing of this and was just waiting for the go-ahead. Uncertain quite what to do, Wilson wrote again to Blatch, seeking guidance on whether the grant had been accepted or not and declaring himself to be "in a quandary with this one."

Also unknown to me at that time was the fact that Zuckerman was in contact with the Chief Medical Officer (CMO), one of the chief architects of UK MMR vaccine policy, Sir Kenneth Calman,[5] informing him that he and his colleagues remained:

> ...very concerned about the unwelcome controversy surrounding the work on Crohn's disease which is carried out at this School by Dr Andrew Wakefield and his group.

Zuckerman reassured Calman that he would stay in touch on this matter with Dr. David Salisbury, the DoH's director of immunization. Ironically, on the very same day that Zuckerman confirmed to the CMO that he would be informing on my activities, I wrote to Zuckerman advising him that because of my concerns about a possible MMR-autism connection, I had proactively arranged a meeting with representatives of the JCVI for the purpose of communicating these concerns. The JCVI is a committee in the UK charged with offering independent advice to the DoH on vaccines and their safety. In recent years, it has been revealed that — far from being independent — many of the committee members have links to various pharmaceutical companies in the forms of grants and consultancies.[6]

Meanwhile, the Royal Free's finance department continued to wrestle with *that check*. Wilson wrote to the medical school accountant, Mr. Tarhan, on February 1, 1997. It was a long, handwritten note confirming that he had received the advice of Blatch who "felt [the medical school] had no option but to accept the funding. He said we should make it clear to Dr A Wakefield that it is done reluctantly because of the contentious nature of his research." Scribbled across the bottom by Tarhan were the telling words:

we spoke since – BAB [Bryan A. Blatch] *will reconsider in view of* **Political overtones**.[7]

Blatch, the medical school secretary, had reversed his position presumably on the instruction of Zuckerman; for "Political" reasons there had been a change of plan. The issues of academic freedom and the children's welfare had been subverted because of "overtones" – including a secret that threatened government interests.

Zuckerman's holy grail – Armstrong's anticipated support for his position from the ethics committee of the BMA – was still awaited. Blatch was designated to nudge it along, and it was he who continued the correspondence with Armstrong. He wrote on February 24, 1997,[8] confirming that the LAB had provided a research grant "to facilitate the setting up of the clinical and scientific study proposed by Dr A Wakefield," the purpose of which was to "search for measles virus in samples obtained from legally aided patients." Dr. Armstrong acknowledged receipt of this letter and confirmed that he would take advice and be in touch shortly.[9]

Meanwhile, blissfully ignorant that I had set the "cat among the pigeons," I was in correspondence with Zuckerman; I had been seeking to answer Zuckerman's question about the government's select committee investigation on vaccines and Crohn's disease. In hindsight, it seems that this claim may have been some kind of strange ruse on the part of Hull to heighten Zuckerman's anxieties and encourage him to move decisively against me. At that time, not privy to the probable reason for Zuckerman's concern over conflict of interest (i.e., that the government stood to be sued), I went on to dispute that on moral, ethical, and scientific grounds no conflict existed in my assisting these children in getting access to the due process of justice.

Zuckerman responded to me, brushing off the matter of the nonexistent select committee[10] as a misunderstanding. He argued again that the funding represented a conflict of interest but did not provide any coherent basis for his position and copied his letter to Armstrong at the BMA,[11] to whom he also wrote:

> I suspect that the legal claim will be on the basis that measles vaccine and the combined MMR may cause Crohn's disease and inflammatory bowel disease and the safety of these preparations has not been established. Expert opinion and the advice of WHO and JCVI is that there is no confirmed evidence of an association with immunisation against measles (and rubella and mumps) and inflammatory bowel disease and that the epidemiological data are flawed.

> While I would not wish to attempt to balance the arguments for academic freedom and the public interest with respect to the protection of children against infection, the position of the medical school is difficult. Further I am deeply concerned by the unconventional funding of research work by interested lawyers acting on behalf of children with inflammatory bowel disease.

Knowing nothing at this time of Zuckerman's correspondence with Armstrong at the BMA, I wrote back to him reaffirming my position and seeking to reassure him that the LAB study would be handled like any other research project. The filed copy of this letter bears Zuckerman's words in the date stamp:

> This does confirm my worst fears.

Armstrong's long awaited response arrived on Zuckerman's desk on March 26, 1997. It would be an understatement to say that it was neither what he had hoped for, nor expected. The letter ran to three pages and carried a resounding message. Armstrong identified the central ethical question as

...whether the research project was scientifically sound and has been approved by an ethics committee... The question of whether health professionals may be involved in litigation is a matter to be borne in mind with regard to publication or use of data but should not determine whether the research itself is in a valid project.

He pointed out the obvious ethical requirements that

"...there should be full and informed consent from the parents of children," and that *"their confidential information should be protected."*

Interestingly, and in complete accordance with my approach since 1992, Armstrong advised that

...the Department of Heath should be informed [of the findings] *in good time.*

On the matter of research funded by the LAB, the letter went on to state, quite bluntly, that it was

...quite logical for the Legal Aid Board, as a publicly funded body to fund research on relevant issues in law, using government money essentially to sue other government departments. Independently conducted research may establish whether or not they have case a in law and is no different from commissioning a medical expert to provide a view.

One question that had taxed Zuckerman — the funding of research where there was a "clear financial interest in the outcome" — was dealt with succinctly: Armstrong wrote,

...funding of research by special interest groups is commonplace and as long as the findings, or uses to which the data is put, are not influenced by the wishes of the funders, this should not be problematic.

As a final slap in the face to Zuckerman, Armstrong concluded that

...to delay or decline to conduct research which appears to be in the public interest on the grounds that it may embarrass the government or a particular health facility does not appear to be a sound moral argument.

Zuckerman had shot himself in the foot. For his part, Armstrong finished by adding a little salt to Zuckerman's angry wound:

...whereas I do not imagine these comments solve your problems I hope we can indicate that a detailed protocol needs to be developed outlining the main ethical and practical issues at each stage... not only for these patients but for many others who may come forward later.

Zuckerman had waited for 6 months for a reply that had effectively blown his case. In the event that Armstrong's response fell into my hands, it would not only derail his plans for putting an end to scientific scrutiny of MMR vaccine at the Royal Free, but would actually be used to endorse the ethical imperative for undertaking such research. In contrast with his anticipated armor-plated endorsement from Armstrong to stop a financial and political threat to the British government, Zuckerman had received what amounted to a reprimand from the BMA.

Zuckerman managed a short but gracious response, thanking the BMA for their "helpful comments" and indicating that he would now explore the issues with the local ethics committee at the hospital. He duly did so but not before he had placed Armstrong's letter at the back of a deep, dark drawer where presumably he hoped it would remain forever, and where (metaphorically) it did remain until the GMC investigation in 2004 caused it to be disclosed.

The BMA's message was clear: not to conduct valid research for political reasons would be unethical. Despite this and without ever disclosing any details, Zuckerman regularly made reference to their authoritative advice in a way that caused me to infer that the BMA shared his concerns about the work and its source of funding. The categoric advice of the UK medical profession's ethics experts was not, however, going to deflect his efforts to stop my research from going ahead on his watch.

Zuckerman turned his attention to the local ethics committee at the Royal Free Hospital. He wrote to the chairman, Dr. Michael Pegg, on April 2, 1997.[12] In the light of what we now know, the letter was quite simply bizarre. Remember how Zuckerman had sent me off on a futile quest for a select committee that did not exist and then wrote to tell me that there was, in fact, no such select committee? Well, it would appear that he continued this ruse with Pegg, adding political gravitas to his concerns by implying some threat to the medical school. He wrote:

Professor Sir David Hull, Chairman of the JCVI wrote to me in February 1997 that Dawbarns solicitors had made a submission to the House of Commons Select Committee that they are working with Mr Wakefield of the Royal Free investigating Crohn's.

When it came to the BMA's advice, it was as if it had all been just a bad dream, the details of which were best forgotten. Zuckerman acknowledged that he had received their advice, but he kept that advice to himself. He reiterated some of the same concerns to Pegg with which the BMA had already comprehensively dealt:

"The dilemma which the School faces is whether it is ethical for lawyers to fund a particular piece of research where a specific action in law is contemplated rather than a scientifically-based research project." Professor Zuckerman continued, asking Dr. Pegg, *"Was it ethical for lawyers to fund research where a specific action in law was contemplated? It has been suggested that I explore with you whether the committee considered these issues."*

His letter ended reassuringly:

...the Medical School does not question the scientific validity of the project, the independence of the research, the academic freedom of the staff and publication in learned scientific journals.

Zuckerman, a virologist and head of the medical school, had not questioned the scientific validity of the research project. In the context of the advice from the BMA's ethics committee as per Armstrong's letter, with an ethical and moral wind at my back, my position should have been unassailable. Pegg responded to Zuckerman on April 15, 1997,[13] stating that he was not aware of any LAB funding. He asked if I had made a false statement to the ethics committee. Zuckerman responded by return:[14]

...there is absolutely no suggestion of any misconduct by Dr Andrew Wakefield.

Zuckerman reiterated laboriously that the issue was an ethical matter on "a possible conflict of interest and data protection in the event of litigation." These letters were never sent to me. I knew nothing of this exchange. No question was ever raised with me by either Pegg or Zuckerman throughout this entire period although it would have been an easy matter for either of them to have asked me, and for me to have answered their questions. I had made my position clear to Zuckerman; there were no secrets from my perspective, and I would have been happy for these discussions to have taken place. But in Zuckerman's furtive game, this might have meant showing his hand, that is, Armstrong's opinion, and that was not about to happen. That was where the matter rested in the spring of 1997.

As became commonplace with the witnesses providing statements to the GMC in their prosecution, Pegg's position had changed by 2005 and was altogether more critical. Although he had been asked specific questions by Zuckerman at the material time and had declined to "assist" with his dilemma, when interviewed by the GMC lawyers, Pegg stated: "In retrospect I believe the failure to disclose the existence of the legal action was a material non disclosure." In fact, in 1996, there was no requirement for such a disclosure. As it turned out, Pegg's concern was based upon the mistaken belief that the LAB funds had been paid directly to me and were being administered from my "back pocket." He went on to make it clear in his oral testimony before the GMC in 2007 that if the funds had been administered by the Special Trustees and, therefore, approved by them, then he would have needed no further knowledge of their provenance since they would have been appropriately vetted and legitimized. Since this is exactly what did happen, as far as Pegg and the Royal Free ethics committee were concerned, I had acted appropriately.

By May 1997, I had grown tired of the whole fiasco over the LAB funding and decided to seek funding elsewhere. Exasperated, I asked the finance department to return the funds in full to the lawyers. Tarhan, head of finance, wrote a memo to Zuckerman and Blatch[15] explaining this. But at the eleventh hour, there was a change of heart without which these essays might never have been written – history could have been very different. As it was, at the bottom of that memo in Zuckerman's writing are the words:

> *Transferred to Special Trustees. They are aware of the situation and the overspend? Discuss with Martin Else*

Thus, it was that the LAB grant, deemed too ethically and politically challenging to be administered by the medical school, was acceptable to be handled by an account managed by a hospital charity for the purposes of conducting valid and ethical research. Perhaps troubled by some vague moral angst, the dean — although he was to deny it later under oath before the GMC — had allowed the research to go ahead, while seemingly washing the medical school's hands of the deed.

In 2007 at the GMC, Zuckerman's memory of events proved fickle, even when jogged by the contemporaneously documented facts. In his evidence, he blundered into one carefully prepared trap after another, eventually threatening to walk out and get his own lawyer. At one stage, when asked how the LAB grant came to be transferred to the Special Trustees account he said:[16]

> Dr Wakefield was consulted. He said return it to the solicitors. Why it was not returned to the solicitors I have no idea but it would have stopped the matter in its tracks, right there and then. Subsequently it was referred to the Special Trustees of the hospital.

Apparently referring to the GMC's prosecution of me and my colleagues he continued:

> If it had been returned to Dawbarns none of this would have materialised.

This comment is telling: if the LAB-funded study of potentially vaccine-damaged children had been successfully stopped in its tracks, would the British government have dodged a bullet and the GMC witch-hunt have then become unnecessary?

Zuckerman was then asked by my senior counsel, Mr. Kieran Coonan, QC, about the memo dealing with the transfer of the check:

> Q: At the bottom of the page, is that your writing?
>
> A: It is my writing, yes.
>
> Q: It looks as if therefore a scheme or arrangement was entered into whereby the money was then to be transferred to the Special Trustees at the hospital.
>
> A: Well, to put this in context, I met with Mr Tarhan to discuss this and he informed me that this was transferred to the Special Trustees. He told me that they were aware of the situation and I also made a note that although Mr Tarhan was very concerned about the overspend by Dr Wakefield, I noted that but I also made an issue of whether to discuss it with Mr Else. The fact that it was transferred to the Special Trustees was not known to me until my attention was drawn to this by the finance officer, Mr Tarhan.

In fact, **it was Zuckerman himself who had signed the check**[18] that enabled the transfer of these funds. It could not have happened without his authority or his signature. Given his volatile emotional state at the GMC hearing, the check was not presented to him in evidence by my senior counsel, Mr. Kieran Coonan, QC. This moment of legal drama was denied to the assembled company.

Although Zuckerman had known of the potential liability of the British government for MMR vaccine damage back in 1996, it was some time before I was given this same message. However, this was to come from a very different source and for a very different reason.

Endnotes

[1] "The Sunday Times has now established that four, probably five, of these children were covered by the legal aid study. And Wakefield had been awarded up to £55,000 to assist their case by finding scientific evidence of a link. Wakefield did not tell his colleagues or medical authorities of this conflict of interest either during or after the research." Deer B. (2004, February 22). Revealed: MMR research scandal. *The Sunday Times.*

[2] GMC vs. Wakefield, Walker-Smith, and Murch. Evidence of Professor Arie Zuckerman. Tr. 15: p. 4.

> **Smith** [prosecution counsel]: *Do you recall, Professor – and please tell us if you do not – whether you knew who the firm of solicitors Dawbarns was in that letter and whether you picked up on it at the time?*

> **Zuckerman:** *I certainly picked up on it at the time. The actual timing is very difficult because I heard about this firm of solicitors from at least two different sources, one was the Department of Health and the other one was by letter from **Professor Sir David Hull**, so it is difficult for me to say chronologically when was the first time that I heard about it unless I see all the documents together, but I was certainly aware of the involvement of a group of solicitors and it did give rise to a lot of concern.* (emphasis added)

And Day 16:

> Q: *You had become aware by this stage that the Legal Aid Board had provided funding through a firm of solicitors representing Crohn's disease sufferers. Where did you get that information from?*

> A: *As I recall it, I received it from the Department of Health and from **Professor Sir David Hull**.* (emphasis added)

> Q: *When you say the Department of Health, any particular person at the Department of Health?*

> A: *I think it will be difficult for me to say that because, as you probably know, I have been an adviser to the Department of Health continuously for 38 years and, therefore, I had numerous contacts there. It could well have been either **Dr Jeremy Metters or Dr Salisbury**, I am not sure who.* (emphasis added)

[3] Zuckerman to Armstrong, Letter. October 11, 1996.

[4] Zuckerman to Wakefield, Letter. March 13, 1997.

[5] Zuckerman to Calman. Letter. January 22, 1997.

[6] Child Health Safety (2009, March 8). UK Government Hands Drug Industry Control of Childhood Vaccination. Message posted to http://childhealthsafety.wordpress.com/2009/03/08/pharma-decide-uk-vaccination/.

[7] Emphasis added.

[8] Brian Blatch to Armstrong at BMA. Letter. February 24, 1997.

[9] Armstrong to Brian Blatch. Letter. February 27, 1997.

[10] Zuckerman to Wakefield. Letter. March 13, 1997.

[11] Zuckerman to Armstrong. Letter. March 13, 1997.

[12] Zuckerman to Michael Pegg. Letter. April 2, 1997.

[13] Pegg to Zuckerman. Letter. April 15, 1997.

[14] Zuckerman to Pegg. Letter. April 17, 1997.

[15] Tarhan to Zuckerman and Blatch. Letter. May 20, 1997.

[16] GMC vs Wakefield, Walker-Smith and Murch. Zuckerman's evidence. Tr. 15 & 16.

[17] In 1997 while expressing his concern about such conflict with regard to LAB funding for a scientific study, Zuckerman wrote an editorial for the *New England Journal of Medicine (NEJM)* strongly supporting universal use of hepatitis B vaccination of the world's infants. At that time, he was a named inventor on a patent related to the hepatitis B vaccine and, as such, might have stood to benefit financially from the policy endorsed in his editorial. At the time, in 1996, strict rules existed for the *NEJM* barring patent holders from writing editorials.

[18] Picture of check available at www.callous-disregard.com.

CHAPTER FOUR

The Whistleblower

Whistleblower. [Noun] An employee, former employee, or member of an organization, especially a business or government agency, who reports misconduct to people or entities that have the power and presumed willingness to take corrective action.

Kirsten Limb was a paralegal at the law firm Dawbarn's. On Monday, April 27, 1998, she called me from their Kings Lynn office in a state of considerable excitement. The previous day, she and Barr had traveled to Newcastle to meet in secret with someone who, in several anonymous calls to their office, had referred to himself as a "whistleblower"; no further information had been forthcoming. Newcastle is a considerable journey from Norfolk, particularly on a Sunday when track repairs and double-time pay for railway staff can drag out a journey to seeming eternity. At exactly noon at the coffee shop on Platform 2 of Newcastle station, they met with "George." "George" was an assumed name and the only one by which he would be identified. He was, apparently, neat and nervous – every inch a civil servant. (Kirsten's attendance notes documenting George's disclosures are provided in italics on pages 66-72.)

George claimed that he was acting on behalf of a colleague – a senior medical officer in the Scottish Office, which is part of the UK government (apparently George himself was a very high ranking civil servant, although his position was not explained). In fact, George and his medical officer "friend" were one and the same, a detail that was disclosed at a second meeting also at Newcastle station 1 year later.[1]

George had moved to the UK from Canada, where he had worked as a principal program immunization advisor in Ontario and was closely involved with the MMR vaccination program. He had been actively recruited to join the Scottish Office as a senior medical officer, particularly to advise on evolving UK MMR vaccination policy.

At that time, a brand of the MMR vaccine had been withdrawn in Canada because it was unsafe; Canada had introduced an MMR vaccine containing the Urabe AM-9 mumps virus (*Trivirix*) in 1986.[2] It soon became apparent that this vaccine caused unacceptably high rates of meningitis.[3] George was invited to sit on the UK's Joint Committee on Vaccination and Immunisation (JCVI) as its Scottish representative. In Canada, he had collated extensive information about the MMR hazard; therefore, he was in an excellent position to advise the DoH and, particularly, Dr. David Salisbury, the UK's chief MMR strategist,[4] on the introduction of the MMR. George claimed:

> *...he was very cautious not to openly release the damning evidence that he had retained from Canada regarding the safety of the MMR vaccine...*

Apparently, however, his attempts to pass this crucial information on to the members of the JCVI were, to his astonishment, rebutted. George pointed out:

> *Canada had been using the Jeryl Lynn[5] [Merck's mumps strain in their MMR vaccine MMR2] MMR before they started using the Urabe strain. They had a good monitoring system in place and, had no axe to grind about the new Urabe vaccines. Yet despite using the Jeryl Lynn MMR for 15 years, they immediately withdrew Urabe after 6 months, because the surveillance system had picked up the side effects [meningitis].*

At the UK's Department of Health, George and other members of the JCVI expressed their

> *...grave disquiet about public documents being issued which were designed to portray the MMR vaccine as 'totally safe' when clearly, it was not.*

George felt:

> *...it was madness to use a vaccine which was unproven.*

He made this point strongly to the JCVI in late spring of 1988. His superiors on the JCVI apparently rejected his advice.

When the decision was taken to introduce MMR in the UK, SmithKline French-Beecham (SKFB), as the British company was apparently then called, did not have a licensed product in the UK. In fact, their own Urabe-containing MMR vaccine, sold under the name of *Trivirix*, was withdrawn in Canada for safety reasons in July 1998, in the *same* month that the *same* vaccine under a different name (*Pluserix*) was granted a license in the UK. On the other hand, Merck Sharp & Dohme (MSD) had a safer MMR vaccine (MMR II) containing the Jeryl Lynn strain of mumps that had been sold for many years in the US without reports of meningitis.[6] However, Merck's vaccine was expensive since, as George put it,

> ...they had to recover their costs.

George explained:

> It was this that promoted the introduction of the Pluserix vaccine, as a competitor to encourage MSD to lower their prices.

Ominously, having withdrawn *Trivirix* in Canada, SmithKline Beecham (SKB) simply repackaged the identical vaccine ingredients as *Pluserix* for use in the UK, apparently irrespective of the risk to children,

> "...there was a determination to sell a [cheaper] MMR vaccine from SmithKline French Beecham [sic]," a British company.

George stressed:

> ...at the time they announced the MMR vaccination campaign, Pluserix was not actually licensed to be used in [the UK]. Nonetheless, the Government had certainly internally announced that it was going to be used and its licensing procedure was rushed through on a 'fast track' basis... safety trials were circumvented to allow the [Pluserix] vaccine to be licensed and widely used.

Again, ominously, George expressed:

> ...absolutely no doubt that short cuts were taken.[7]

But there was a "problem," as George put it:

> ...introduction of the MMR vaccine in the United Kingdom had been delayed for four months because SmithKline French Beecham [sic] were very reluctant to obtain a license for the product in the United Kingdom. They were aware of the safety concerns based on the experience in Canada and Japan in particular, and were extremely concerned about their liability.

The key to the mystery of Zuckerman's fears for the British government, as outlined in Chapter 3, "The Dean's Dilemma," may lie in the manner in which the UK vaccine manufacturer's concerns were dealt with. George continued:

> It would appear that a legal waiver was offered between Smith Kline French Beecham [sic] and the Department of Health ...the manufacturers were very concerned about trying to obtain a license for the MMR in the United Kingdom, in view of the problems with it in Canada. He [George] and his colleagues felt that the manufacturers, being very astute and having their own legal advisors, would have had some sort of agreement in writing about their liability.

This was confirmed when George raised the issue with a female representative of what had then become SmithKline Beecham. She responded with the words,

> we are immunising the children and the Government is immunising us.

He took this as confirmation that a deal had been struck whereby the government had assumed SKB's liability for damage to children arising out of the high-risk strategy of using *Pluserix* vaccine. Unknowingly, the taxpayer was on the hook for a "dirty" vaccine.

And concerns about liability were not confined to SKB; George pointed out that the question of legal liability over the use of an unsafe vaccine had been raised at the JCVI since, as he put it,

> Members of the committee were anxious about their own status bearing in mind the warnings that [George] had given.

How could such a situation have arisen? George informed Barr and Limb that

> ...the JCVI was envisaged as being a committee with an entirely advisory role. However, they were acting beyond this brief. There were a small number of 'hard core' members of the JCVI who were absolutely not interested [about safety concerns] and were really political animals.

Influence over the committee's proceedings appears to have been exerted by this "hard core" in part by controlling access to information. George explained:

...whenever there was a meeting of the JCVI, the minutes of the meeting were always about 6 months late in being circulated.

It appears that committee members received, as George put it, these "very sanitized" minutes just the day before the next meeting. Limb's attendance note captured the disquiet among some JCVI members over the committee's decision-making process.

When [George] mentioned his concerns about the [MMR] vaccine and brought the information he had to the attention of the committee (including medical literature etc that had come to his attention on Ontario) some JCVI members expressed concerns and wanted more information... these members were seriously concerned and asking repeatedly for caution and for further information to be supplied. However, because these minutes of meetings were six months late in circulating, decisions were being implemented [by the "hard core"] before information had come through.

George insisted that there must be internal documents detailing this. He continued,

Worries were discussed at the meetings, but again the minutes of the meeting down-played this.

George indicated that he had retained many relevant documents, although he felt sure that many of those held at the DoH would have been illegally destroyed. While the government had made it a major offense for civil servants to destroy evidence in this way, George admitted:

...they could not really stop it going on.

George also said that there was a big row about the change in contraindications to the vaccine and that certain members of the JCVI felt that millions of British children had been used in "one big experiment." He confirmed that once the government was beyond the token clinical trials involving these children,

...the next decision was to implement the MMR vaccine.

George went on to identify the individuals whom he considered to be culpable. The medical secretariat of the JCVI was singled out. The secretariat was responsible for the minutes of meetings and, therefore, controlled information. He described one senior member as "a very driven man" and "an exceptionally arrogant man… determined to get himself up the ladder." But, apparently, the problems were not confined to one person. George claimed that

> …in fact the whole environment in public health at that time was bordering on the fascist.

He identified certain members of the Scottish Office and the Ministry of Health whom he claimed

> …were very rabidly right wing. This was the character of these offices at the time.

George continued by warning Barr, Limb, and me that

> …some of the key people in this may not stop at anything.

So despite being brought in to advise on the introduction of MMR in the UK, George's expert concerns were ignored. In fact, the high risk *Pluserix* vaccine was to take the lion's share of the UK MMR market. In light of its known dangers, one would have expected that vigilant surveillance of adverse events would have been put in place. George and the rest of the Scottish Committee strongly advocated for such surveillance and

> …pressed for an increase in funding to allow more active surveillance.

Active surveillance (as opposed to passive surveillance, which is awaiting spontaneous reports of adverse reactions from doctors) involves the prospective ascertainment of adverse reactions through active canvassing of data from primary care doctors. George was involved in trying to set up some sort of surveillance system, but no money was given to him to do this. According to George, the money had to come through a senior member of the medical secretariat who controlled millions of pounds to implement the vaccination program but was very resistant to spending any money on monitoring safety. George continued to try to press this person for funds in order to provide adequate surveillance of side effects, but despite his repeated efforts, this was denied.

The rest of the story was, inevitably, a rewrite of the Canadian, Japanese, and Australian experiences. As increasing numbers of reports of meningitis following *Pluserix* immunization came in, George described how

...eventually other members of the JCVI began to realise what was happening, and began putting increasing pressure on Salisbury, to look more closely at adverse events after MMR. Salisbury gave a very small amount of money to the Public Health Laboratory Service (PHLS), really expecting them to prove that there was no problem with the vaccine. Instead, as we know, they found problems. The whole thing blew up over a weekend, and Pluserix had to be withdrawn. Salisbury had to fly to the United States on Saturday of that weekend, and go to see Merck Sharp Dohme senior management. He had to go 'cap in hand' and ask them to divert some of the worldwide MMR vaccine to the United Kingdom, to cover the enormous gap created by the withdrawal of Pluserix.

George felt strongly that between the years of 1988 and 1992, the clinical indicators of the problem with *Pluserix* were definitely there but were not being noted. It was not just the Scottish Office that was expressing concerns. Various doctors also raised concerns in the UK. George pointed out that, as a damage limitation exercise, one senior medical member

...sought to reassure his colleagues in the JCVI, that the brain inflammation that many of the children were experiencing would not leave any long term effects, and that also any meningitis that developed was "aseptic" [non-bacterial] as though this made it all alright.

In fact, George was convinced that some children suffered permanent damage from *Pluserix*. Prior to his public health career, George disclosed that he

"...had been a paediatrician who specialised in the rehabilitation of brain injured children, so he did have direct experience of the awful situation that parents of children affected by the MMR found themselves in." He appeared to hold *"a very strong view that there should be justice for the children that had been damaged by the vaccine."* Clearly he felt somewhat guilty that *"instead of going to the top and exposing all this, he did not do that at the time, but stayed quiet because he had children to support at University."*

George continued:

"...the present government [Labour] has vowed to improve things, but unfortunately it had inherited the same Civil Servants," presumably with the same interests at heart.

Apparently, in order to ensure continued mutual protection, the week before they left office just before the election, the Conservative government

> ...gave five-year contracts to their Civil Servants that could be enforced if anyone tried to get them out subsequently. In the event they lost the election, the only way for an incoming party to get rid of them would be to give out vast handouts, and then they would be accused of wasting public funds.

One year later George was still struggling with his conscience. At a second meeting – one that I attended and also at Newcastle station – he went over the same ground and confirmed the facts covered in the previous meeting, except that at this second meeting these facts were disclosed in the first person. For that reason, Limb wrote,

> ...what he said carried very much more weight.

He told again how he had repeatedly given direct warnings to senior medical members about the risks over the Urabe-containing MMR vaccine – warnings which they had ignored. I was later able to corroborate the contents of the attendance note taken by Limb. For George, there was a price to pay for his dissent. At the material time, circa 1988, he was in his early 50s, he had two children at university, and

> ...he felt very loyal to the Civil Service and the job he had within it.

He had put himself in a difficult position by criticizing JCVI decisions. According to George, with Dr. Kenneth Calman's move from Scotland to London as the UK's new Chief Medical Officer, he had been next in line for Calman's position in Scotland but had been passed over for this. It was of greater concern to George that he was a signatory to the Official Secrets Act, which forbade him from taking home copies of official documents. He was worried that if it were found out that he had been in breach of this Act, he would likely to go to prison. In her attendance note, Limb documented:

> "He obviously remained very unhappy throughout his time in the Civil Service, grappling with his duty to his family on the one hand and his anxiety over the safety of the vaccines on the other." Elsewhere she noted, "He is obviously a very unhappy man, trapped with an aching conscience and rather terrified at the consequences of what he has done."

He was, not unreasonably, concerned for his own safety. When contacted later, he stated that he did not wish to be the "next David Kelly." Dr. David Kelly was a scientist in the UK's Ministry of Defence who, many believe, was murdered for threatening to disclose the fact that Iraq was not in possession of weapons of mass destruction.[8]

So there, in a railway station café in the far north of England, was somebody who was once one of the most senior medical officials in Scotland, blowing the whistle on, at the very least, the attitude toward safety and children's welfare of some of the UK's top medical officials. He indicated that he was prepared to provide a detailed statement. No one had any doubt at all that he was telling the truth, and there was little doubt that he would be believed should he come before a court or parliamentary select committee despite whatever attempts were made to discredit him. As he had crossed the Rubicon, he acknowledged that there was little point in keeping his identity completely secret. Indeed, Limb considered that he was quite relieved for someone to have known exactly who he was. George's real name is Dr. Alistair Thores. He lives in Edinburgh, Scotland. He would do well to realize sooner rather than later that a whistleblower is much safer once he has gone public in the public interest. If he has ever watched *The Insider*, he will know that information is dangerous only as long as you are the only one who knows it.

There is much more that can and will be written about the Urabe episode. I have confined this chapter to my state of knowledge in 1996-7 since it was the insights provided by George's disclosures that were, in part, my motivation to fight for a **safety first** vaccine policy. This story highlights so many of the problems within the UK's vaccine politburo, not least of which are the disproportionate influence of a few individuals, the apparent manipulation of information and access to it, and above all, where the perception of the importance of vaccine safety ranks in the priorities of those who are charged with looking out for our children. The Urabe episode throws these issues into sharp relief. Against expert advice, a dangerous vaccine was given preferred status. Children were the experimental marketplace. Shortcuts were apparently taken to fast-track the licensing process for this vaccine. Despite warnings, adverse events surveillance operated at a bare minimum on a sort of "if we don't look, we won't see" policy. The UK safety studies lasted only 3 weeks, whereas the Canadians were reporting that in many cases vaccine-induced meningitis didn't even start until after this period.[9] The vaccine manufacturers and JCVI members had reasonable fears that they might be liable, and SKB, for their part, appear to have been given a "Get Out of Jail Free" card by Her Majesty's Government. Confirmation of this was later to appear in the JCVI minutes of May 7, 1993, where it states:

...SKB continue to sell the Urabe MMR without liability.[10]

The vaccine proved to be unsafe for UK children, just as it had for other children around the world. Permanent damage to children was denied and this denial continues. Years later, Salisbury was to deny any knowledge of an indemnity[11] (initially, at least) in spite of the fact that the JCVI minutes are unambiguous and entirely consistent with George's firsthand experience. The matter clearly needs to be resolved, and I suspect there is considerable fear of public scrutiny.

One of the enduring mysteries is the issue of the respective costs of the different MMR vaccines. As Martin Walker noted in "The Urabe Farrago,"[12] JCVI minutes and all other available data recorded how MMR II was 3-4 times more costly than *Pluserix*, but more recent documents identify the MMR II product at £1 in the early catch up phase (when MMR was first introduced) going up to £2 after that, whereas the supply agreement for *Pluserix* records the cost of this vaccine at £3.80 plus tax. Was this high price negotiated as part of the deal?

In 1997, while I sought to bring my safety concerns to the attention of members of the JCVI, behind the scenes these same doctors were running with a parallel agenda. Hull of the JCVI had alerted Zuckerman to my work with Barr; he had seemingly exercised Zuckerman about a nonexistent government select committee, and later sought to question Walker-Smith's clinical care of children and the associated research by making misleading claims about it.[13] Might it be coincidental that Hull was also on the JCVI that was responsible for advising on the use of the *Pluserix* MMR vaccine?

Zuckerman had tried to prevent the Legal Aid Board pilot study on the basis of "conflict of interest," but did not disclose to me that this conflict was the fact that it was the UK government that was (and presumably still is) liable for SKB's[14] MMR vaccine damage.

The gulf between my perception of MMR vaccine safety and that of Salisbury, the head of the UK's immunization program, is exemplified in one of the concluding paragraphs of his statement to the GMC's lawyers:[15]

It is hard to quantify how much the DH has expended financially to deal with this [public concerns over MMR safety]. *Huge resources have been spent in communication initiatives entirely for the purpose of restoring public and professional confidence for* **a vaccine with an exemplary safety record.**[16]

Two of the UK's three licensed brands, introduced in 1988 and withdrawn for safety reasons in 1992 – "exemplary"? The huge resources could have been better spent.

Endnotes

[1] February 28, 1999.

[2] Initially as Institute Armand-Frappier, Quebec, later as SmithKline French-Beecham.

[3] Champagne et al. *Can Dis Weekly Rep.* 1987;13:155-157

[4] Curriculum Vitae of Dr. David Salisbury. Under "personal achievements" it reads: "Strategy design and policy implementation MMR vaccination 1988."

[5] Jeryl Lynn was the name of Dr. Maurice Hilleman's daughter from whom this mumps strain was isolated. Hilleman was in charge of Merck's vaccine program.

[6] See Martin Walker's article titled "The Urabe Farrago." Retrieved from: http://www.wesupportandywakefield.com/documents/The%20Urabe%20Farrago.pdf

[7] There are at least two parts to this: firstly, according to the minutes of the working party to discuss the introduction of MMR vaccine (January 23, 1987), data from other countries (the US and Finland) that used Merck's MMR II that contained the Jeryl-Lynn mumps strain and not the Urabe-containing MMR, were accepted as a proxy for the safety of the Urabe-containing vaccine. Secondly, the UK "trial" of MMR lasted only 3 weeks. Meningitis following the Urabe-containing MMR is rarely seen before 21 days post-vaccination and can occur up to 35 days later. The UK "trial" would have missed it.

[8] Goslett M. (2010, January 25) David Kelly post mortem to be kept secret for 70 years as doctors accuse Lord Hutton of concealing vital information. Retrieved from: http://www.dailymail.co.uk/news/article-1245599/David-Kelly-post-mortem-kept-secret-70-years-doctors-accuse-Lord-Hutton-concealing-vital-information.html

[9] See also endnote number 7 for this chapter.

[10] JCVI minutes of May 7, 1993.

[11] Salisbury denies knowledge of indemnity for any manufacturer of MMR: "As has been stated on innumerable occasions, there was no immunity/indemnity given to MMR manufacturers." E-mail from David Salisbury to Clifford Miller, September 13, 2006.

[12] See Martin Walker's article titled "The Urabe Farrago," page 22, footnote 34. Retrieved from: http://www.wesupportandywakefield.com/documents/The%20Urabe%20Farrago.pdf

[13] Hull letter to Zuckerman about MRC presentation "Since these children have no evidence of chronic inflammatory bowel disease." July 6, 1998. This is false.

[14] Now Glaxo SmithKline.

[15] GMC vs Wakefield, Walker-Smith, and Murch. Statement of Dr. David Salisbury. September 20, 2006; page 29, paragraph 150.

[17] Emphasis added.

CHAPTER FIVE

Ethics and the Masses

Informed consent is a crucial element of the foundation upon which ethical medical practice rests. Providing patients, parents, or guardians with an honest assessment of the risks and benefits of any medical procedure requires the physician to be, to the best of his or her ability, "informed."[1]

While sitting in the chamber of the General Medical Council (GMC), accused of ethical violations in the investigation of *The Lancet 12* and irresponsible scaremongering about MMR vaccine safety, I was listening to the earnest testimony of the UK's DoH Director of Immunisation, Dr. David Salisbury; it was at this point that I determined that this brief essay should go on the record. It relates to a mass vaccination campaign using an experimental vaccine combination – measles and rubella (MR) – that was administered to approximately 8 million UK school children[2] over a 1-month period in November 1994. The justification for the campaign was a mathematically-predicted measles epidemic. The principal architects of the campaign were Salisbury and his boss, Dr. Kenneth Calman, the UK's Chief Medical Officer. Through an intense and frightening advertising campaign,[3] parents were motivated to get their children revaccinated by the threat of up to 50 deaths from measles.

There are well-established side effects from measles-containing vaccines (MCV); anaphylaxis is one of these. Anaphylaxis refers to a rapidly developing and potentially serious allergic reaction that affects a number of different areas of the body at one time. Severe anaphylactic reactions can be fatal, and the public is well aware of deaths in children with peanut allergy following inadvertent exposure. While many people experience allergy symptoms only as a minor annoyance, a minority of allergic people are susceptible to a reaction that can lead to shock (a dramatic reduction in blood pressure) and even death.

Anaphylaxis is often triggered by substances (allergens) that are injected (such as MCV) or ingested and thereby gain access into the bloodstream. An explosive reaction involving the skin, lungs, nose, throat, and gastrointestinal tract can then result. Although severe cases of anaphylaxis can occur within seconds or minutes of exposure and be rapidly fatal if untreated, many reactions can be ended with prompt medical therapy.

Anaphylaxis is likely to be more common and more serious with second and subsequent exposures to an allergen since the body's immune system has been primed by the initial exposure and is capable of reacting more vigorously.

The best and safest way to deal with anaphylaxis is to (1) be fully informed of the risk; that is, be aware of the possibility that anaphylaxis is a side effect of the exposure; (2) avoid exposure to the offending allergen if there is any history of a prior reaction; and (3) have access to immediate treatment such as epinephrine (adrenalin) in the event of this reaction.

As I have already explained, anaphylaxis is a known risk of MCV, and it was predictable — with an absolute certainty — that cases would occur as a consequence of the MR campaign. Therefore, it was essential for the vaccine directorate of the DoH to fully evaluate the relevant medical literature in order to adequately assess the extent of the anaphylaxis risk and to decide how to deal with it when planning this experimental mass vaccination campaign. In order that the DoH might accurately and ethically warn parents and children of this risk and evaluate the risk-benefit ratio of the MR strategy, this comprehensive evaluation of the literature was a prerequisite — failure to do it was not an ethical option. In order to assist in such a risk assessment, doctors in New York in 1992 had reported their experience of five cases of potentially life-threatening anaphylaxis in 2,789 booster doses of MMR — reactions that were aborted by the timely and potentially lifesaving administration of epinephrine (adrenalin) or diphenhydramine.[4] MMR was the common denominator in the vaccines received by the affected individuals. Importantly, these recipients were school-age children, with three being 8, 8, and 9 years old respectively; therefore, according to the prevailing US vaccine schedule, they would have already received at least one MCV.

Without prompt treatment, this reaction, which occurred in 1 in 558 recipients of an MCV, might well have been fatal. The data from New York indicate that anaphylaxis is likely to be more common and more severe in older children who have previously been exposed to an MCV – precisely the children who were targeted in the UK's MR revaccination campaign.[5] For the UK, this figure equated to the potential for up to 14,337 cases of a potentially life-threatening complication in that campaign.

But parents were not warned.

There was no mention of anaphylaxis at all in the information leaflet prepared by the DoH and upon which parents based their consent to vaccination.[6]

To make matters worse, the same information leaflet claimed that reactions were expected to be less likely with the booster dose.[7] I am not aware of any evidence that anaphylaxis is less likely or less severe on re-exposure.[8] The data from New York with MCV boosters would suggest quite the opposite.

The MR campaign was undertaken largely in the nation's schools rather than in doctors' offices. Despite this, family doctors and nurses were sent their own information document by Salisbury's department. The document confirmed that the immunizations would take place in school and that general practitioners would not be supplied with the MR vaccine until after the school-based vaccination program had been completed.

In the information for doctors, under the heading of "Contraindications to MR immunisation"[9] it states clearly that children with a history of anaphylaxis following a measles- or rubella-containing vaccine should not be given the MR vaccine.

In the certain knowledge that anaphylaxis would (and did)[10] occur, and in light of the published evidence that it could occur with a relatively high frequency and that it is potentially fatal unless treated promptly, treatment facilities should, without a doubt, have been available (and known to be by all involved) wherever the vaccine was to be administered. They were not, at least at my children's school or those of any other parent of whom I have inquired.

We shall never know what actually happened. It is my opinion that a state of deliberate ignorance exists. Despite the fact that the MR vaccine had never been used before, despite the fact that the UK had no experience of mass vaccination campaigns, and despite the published risks of a potentially life-threatening reaction, there was no *active* surveillance to determine the true rate of adverse events during the MR campaign. Despite the reliance on the failed system of *passive* surveillance – i.e., receiving spontaneous doctors' reports of suspected adverse reactions – the MR campaign was associated with a high rate of reported adverse reactions. This probably represented no more that 10 percent of the true adverse reactions to an MCV and, based upon the experience of the US

Centers for Disease Control and Prevention, probably considerably less.[11]

For cases of anaphylaxis based upon spontaneous reports, the Joint Committee on Vaccination and Immunisation (JCVI) minutes of May 5, 1995, document that in the MR campaign

...*few cases had been severe or life-threatening.*[12]

Here we have confirmation of the fact that some parents had unwittingly put their children's lives at risk because they had never been told that such risk existed. The concept of *informed consent* appears to have counted for nothing. Adrenalin – sometimes multiple doses — were required to abort some of these attacks.

In a paper endorsing the merits of the MR campaign, Dr. Felicity Cutts[13] reported that with MMR vaccine anaphylaxis occurs in up to 1 in 20,000 doses (i.e., an expected 400 anaphylaxis cases following MR vaccine). This is certainly an underestimate because her data was based, almost exclusively, on inadequate surveilliance methods and primary MMR vaccination of 1 year olds. The observation of Kalat et al. of severe anaphylaxis in 1 in 558 school-age children reinforces the fact that the risk is likely to be considerably greater in older children getting a booster dose.

It is unthinkable that those responsible for writing the information leaflet for parents simply forgot about anaphylaxis, and this is confirmed by the information provided to family doctors. It would have been negligent of them not to have reviewed the literature exhaustively in advance of putting the campaign into effect. Trying to persuade parents of the merits of an MR campaign on the basis of up to 50 possible measles deaths while ethically warning them of the possibility of up to 14,337 anaphylaxis deaths from the MR vaccine would have doomed the campaign to failure. In my opinion, parents were deliberately frightened by a powerful advertising campaign to get their children revaccinated with an experimental vaccine in an untested mass revaccination strategy. The outstanding question is whether or not a deliberate decision was taken not to warn of the risks of anaphylaxis.

I wrote on multiple occasions to Salisbury and Calman, seeking to alert them to my concerns about adverse immune effects of MCV and, in particular, the risks of revaccination, especially in relation to inflammatory bowel disease. At the time, I was unfamiliar with the anaphylaxis issue, but the principles are similar. I sought any evidence that any MCV-revaccination policy had ever been studied for safety but could find none.

As part of this quest, I contacted Dr. Christenson on the basis of her being one of the architects of the Swedish vaccine program. Systematic revaccination with MMR started in Sweden in 1982.[14] I asked her about her expert knowledge of safety studies of 2-dose MMR schedules. She replied:

> I must avow that I don't quite understand what you mean with if there has [sic] been any safety studies of the 2-dose measles vaccine schedule. We have followed the 12-year old children with blood specimens drawn before vaccination and 2 months after vaccination. This is a form of safety study.

Clearly, measurement of serum antibodies following revaccination of 12 year olds is *no* kind of a safety study at all (serum antibodies at 2 months are a measure of short-term vaccine *efficacy*). Christenson later confirmed to me in a telephone call that there had been no safety studies of 2-dose schedules in Sweden, nor was she aware of any having been performed elsewhere, reinforcing the experimental nature of this policy in the UK. Despite the MR campaign having been a mass experiment on human subjects, there is no indication that an ethics committee (EC) approval was ever sought or granted.

How does this rank, in my opinion, in the great scheme of ethical violations? At the GMC I was found guilty of not having EC approval for having a sample of blood taken from my own children and several of their friends at my son's birthday party with full and informed consent from the children and their parents. The blood samples were taken for comparison with those from children with autism. The blood was taken by a suitably qualified medical practitioner with standard aseptic precautions. Children were rewarded with the equivalent of just over $7. The entire procedure passed off without mishap or complaint. This process did not have the approval of an EC, which I now accept was naïve, but it was most certainly *not* unethical. In contrast, the MR campaign had multiple ethical failings on many levels, but the most staggering omission of all seems to me to have been the failure to alert parents to the known threat of severe adverse reactions – to deny them the fundamental right of informed consent in making a decision about their child. It puts the *birthday party* into the shade and rather makes a mockery of the post-GMC headlines about my callous disregard.

Endnotes

[1] Wakefield AJ, Blaxill M, Haley B, Ryland A, Hollenbeck D, Johnson J, Moody J, Stott C. Response to Dr. Ari Brown and the Immunization Action Coalition. *Medical Veritas*. 2009;6:1907-1924.

[2] Cutts F. Revaccination against measles and rubella. *BMJ*. 1996;312:589-590.

[3] Minutes of JCVI meeting May 5, 1995; 6.5 para 2. *HEA measles/Rubella campaign report: The HEA* [Health Education Authority] *did acknowledge the view that the TV advert used had been a little frightening, and also that not enough information on the possible side-effects of the vaccine had been provided for some people.*

[4] Kalet A, Berger DK, Bateman WB, Dubitsky J, Covitz K. Allergic reactions to MMR vaccine. *Pediatrics*. 1992;89:168-9.

[5] Cutts F. Revaccination against measles and rubella. *BMJ*. 1996;312:589-590.

[6] JCVI minutes of November 3, 1995. In section 10.1, paragraph 2, it is disclosed that anaphylaxis had not been mentioned in the parents' leaflet."

[7] Measles. Why every child in school needs to be protected from measles this autumn. 1994 Health Education Authority/Department of Health

[8] With the exception of specific desensitization regimes undertaken by experts.

[9] Measles and Rubella Immunization Campaign. PL CMO(94)12/PL CMO(94)15 September 27 1994. Page 4.

[10] JCVI minutes of January 27, 1995. Section 6.7, paragraph 2.

[11] Rosenthal S, Chen R. The Reporting Sensitivities of Two Passive Surveillance Systems for Vaccine Adverse Events. *Am J Public Health*. 1995;85:1706-1709.

[12] JCVI minutes of May 5, 1995. Section 6.7.

[13] Cutts F. Revaccination against measles and rubella. *BMJ*. 1996;312:589-590.

[14] Bottiger M, Christenson B, Romanus V, Taranger J, Starndell A. Swedish experience of two dose vaccination programme aiming at eliminating measles, mumps, and rubella. *BMJ*. 1987;295:1264-1267.

[15] Letter from Dr. B. Christenson to AJW, referred to also in paper Wakefield AJ and Montgomery SM. Measles, mumps, rubella vaccine: through a glass, darkly. *Adverse Drug Reactions & Toxicological Reviews*. 2000;19:265-283.

CHAPTER SIX

The Dean's Press Briefing

By winter 1997, the *case series* paper had been accepted for publication in *The Lancet*. In view of some advance publicity and the growing controversy that surrounded the vaccine issue in particular, it was considered likely that the paper would attract considerable interest from the media.

Since his appointment as dean, Zuckerman saw media attention as being a positive thing for a medical school that had been becalmed in the academic doldrums for some years. In order to "court" news outlets and gain attention for the medical school, an entity known as the Media Group had been formed under Zuckerman's chairmanship and included members of both the medical school and the hospital as well as Phillipa Hutchinson, the school's press officer.

As dean and chairman of the media group, Zuckerman made the decision to hold a press briefing on the forthcoming *Lancet* publication, timed for the day before the study appeared in print. While this decision was influenced by a 1995 press briefing on Crohn's disease and its possible link to measles vaccination, Zuckerman and Hutchinson were later to express opinions that were polar opposites on the outcome of that prototype press briefing.

I approached the idea of a press briefing with some anxieties; by this stage, I had examined the issue of MMR vaccine safety in great detail. I had reviewed all of the published scientific literature about measles and MMR vaccine safety studies on the basis that, as part of investigating parental concerns and before calling into question MMR vaccine safety, it was essential to have done so. On a personal level, I was dismayed that I hadn't done this research before vaccinating my two older children. On a global level, it was clear that the safety studies had been wholly inadequate. "George" the whistleblower had major concerns about the attitude of many of his public health colleagues toward concerns over vaccine safety. The forced withdrawal of MMR vaccines that had been "spun" as being *completely safe* was testament to their failings. In the light of these concerns and the forthcoming publicity, I wrote to my colleagues

5 weeks before publication, informing them of my position with respect to a media statement on MMR vaccination.

Re: MMR and Autistic Enteropathy: Forthcoming publicity[1]

Firstly, the paper has been officially accepted by The Lancet after some minor revisions. They will be sending proofs next week and I will pass one on to each of the authors.

I felt that in view of the imminent publicity regarding our work, it was important to write and clarify my own position. Clearly, pending a press-briefing or other communications with the press, which now seems inevitable, we need to have considered our points of view, well in advance of publication. There may be points upon which we disagree, but I do not think that this is a problem, as long as that is made clear. If we can both recognize and respect each other's position, then there should be no ambiguity. I have thought about this issue almost continuously over the last 5 years, firstly in a relationship to inflammatory bowel disease, and latterly autistic enteropathy, and I have tried to set this out below, as a template for more detailed discussion.

In addition to our own work and that of others, my opinion is also based upon a comprehensive review of all safety studies performed on measles, MR and MMR vaccines and re-vaccination policies. This now runs into a report compiled by me of some 250 pages, which I am happy to let you see. In summary, the safety studies are derisory, and appear to reflect sequential assumptions about measles vaccine safety, MMR safety and latterly, two dose vaccine safety, where each assumption has potentially compounded the dangers inherent in the first.

*In view of this, if my opinion is sought, I cannot support the continued use of the **polyvalent**[3] MMR vaccine. I have no doubt of the value of the continued use of the **monovalent**[4] vaccines, and will continue to support their use until the case has been proven one way or another of the measles link to chronic inflammatory bowel disease. I believe that 1998 will see some conclusive data in favour of the measles link from both our own work and the USA. I recommend that measles vaccination is deferred in children with a strong family history of IBD.[5]*

Paradoxically, attempts to sustain credence in MMR safety by quoting data from a surveillance scheme that is widely recognized to be inadequate, and to dismiss parents' claims of a link between their child's disorder and MMR without due investigation, in breach of the most fundamental rules of clinical medicine, is unacceptable. The failure of the regulatory authorities to honour their commitments to MMR vaccine safety has created a House-of-Cards that threatens all vaccine policies.

When parents have their claims dismissed, out of hand ...[6] they create frustration, resentment and distrust; similarly disaffected parents form into self help groups such as AIA and JABS, many of the members of which are articulate and well-read. Their anger is compounded as the case-numbers grow and their anxieties go unheeded. Finally Doctors such as us, perceive a pattern to the disease and its links with the MMR that becomes self-evident. When the data are presented, the anger of many parents boils over, the press has a field day, and the House of Cards crashes to the ground.

Loss of trust in the regulatory authorities is inevitable and vaccination compliance, across the board, is affected – a difficult and dangerous situation. There is no doubt in my mind that responsibility for this volatile state of affairs rests, not with us, but firmly upon the shoulders of the policy makers; that is, the JCVI and the Department of Health. They have started from the position that the MMR vaccine is safe, and that any change in the policy following claims of adverse events, must be set against that position. Their starting point was, and remains, wrong. Any drug, and especially one that involves 3 live viruses, must be considered dangerous until proven otherwise: this has never been proven and, therefore, all claims of adverse events should have been thoroughly investigated. They have failed to honour this obligation.

In an attempt to avert the House-of-Cards collapsing, I will strongly recommend the use of **monovalent**[7] vaccines as opposed to the polyvalent vaccines. This will not compromise children by increasing their risk of wild infection, and may reduce the risk of apparent synergy between the component viruses that have been identified by Dr. Scott Montgomery as a risk factor for inflammatory bowel disease, and may well be a risk for autism in our children, currently under investigation.

I appreciate that you cannot (or may feel that you cannot) support this stance, and I completely respect that. I value your opinion and your friendship.

Zuckerman was copied in on this letter. My position on MMR was made crystal clear, and the reasons for that position had been laid out. Zuckerman replied on January 22, 1998, saying:

> *You kindly sent me a copy of your letter of 15th January addressed to your senior colleagues stating your own position with regard to MMR and your various studies... I venture to make the following comments in my capacity as a virologist with considerable experience in vaccine development and evaluation. You support the continued use of the **monovalent**[4] vaccines and you write that you have no doubt of their value. To my knowledge this has not been repeated by the media... It is vital, in your own interest and that of children, that you clearly state your support for **monovalent**[4] vaccination.*

For reasons that are uncertain, both my initial letter to colleagues and Zuckerman's response were missing from Zuckerman's disclosures to the GMC lawyers during the preparation of their case against me.

The transcript of the GMC hearing, read verbatim, is a lesson in how to land a fish without putting too much of a bend on the rod. During cross-examination, Kieran Coonan, QC, my senior counsel, led Zuckerman into the circumstances of the press briefing:

> **Coonan:** *There had been something of a track record of holding press conferences or press briefings at the Royal Free. There had been one following the publication of the paper by Dr Wakefield in 1995.*
>
> **Zuckerman:** *That is correct.*
>
> **Coonan:** *That was following the publication of a paper involving Crohn's disease.*
>
> **Zuckerman:** *That is correct.*
>
> **Coonan:** *That appeared to be a successful model and obviously was thought to reflect well on the school.*
>
> **Zuckerman:** *I am sorry, no. It did not reflect well on the school at all because the result of that press conference was an almost dramatic fall in immunisation against measles because, once again, the measles vaccine was blamed for this. The press, of course, found this a very exciting story. It was not a model of a press briefing and*

we had cause to regret that it took the turn of event... It was not a model press briefing; it was a disaster.

In her statement to the GMC, Hutchinson, the press officer, had painted an altogether different picture:

I do recall the team being pleased with the quality of the coverage as it had conveyed the complexities of the science and given a balanced view. As the first press briefing was a success, and due to the overwhelming advance publicity it was decided to hold another press briefing. It would have been the dean [Zuckerman] who decided to hold a press briefing.

Referring back to the 1995 briefing in cross examination, Coonan asked Zuckerman the obvious question:

Coonan: *If that was so bad in your eyes, why did you allow the one in 1998 to go ahead?*

Zuckerman: *It is not a question of me allowing. There is a media group which is shared between the hospital and the Medical School. I, as the Dean of the Medical School, simply chaired that committee. What was agreed by the media group was that the changes in the bowels of children with autism, the pathological changes, were important significant new findings. I, with the rest of the media group, agreed that this should be subject to a press briefing for two reasons: we were aware that The Lancet were going to issue a press statement; and, secondly, we felt that it was important that these pathological changes, and no more than those pathological changes, be presented at a press briefing to make sure that they understood the significance of the pathological changes, nothing to do with measles vaccines.*

In fact, as head of the medical school *and* the media group, it *was* Zuckerman's prerogative to decide whether a press briefing took place or not. In the event, he decided that a press briefing was the appropriate way forward. His claim about *The Lancet's* intention to issue a press statement was in error. In fact *The Lancet* never issued a press statement about the paper at the time of its publication, and in evidence, *The Lancet's* editor, Richard Horton, told the GMC that there had never been an intention to do so.

Crucially — and most importantly — never at any stage was there a plan, directive, request, or agreement that the press briefing would make no mention of vaccines and would be confined to the pathological changes, that is, the intestinal disease in autistic children. There is absolutely no documentary evidence to support this and plenty that refutes it. Hutchinson's statement provides an insight into the dean's state of mind at the material time. She wrote:

> *The aim was... to ensure that the public knew that opinion [on the MMR] among the authors was not uniform. It appeared to me that the authors were at one in respect of the scientific findings [bowel disease] but not in respect of the wider implications [for vaccination]. The Dean wanted this to come across... I remember that a key concern of his was to make it clear that there was a diversity of opinion among the authors of the Lancet paper; another was to ensure that journalists realised that the school fully supported government policy on immunisation.*[8]

Hutchinson's recollection was identical to mine and, while I was not part of the media group, I was bound to act on their instruction. The dean's earnest position that the briefing was to be "nothing to do with measles vaccines" was off to a bad start. Coonan pressed Zuckerman further on his motive for holding a press briefing:

> **Coonan:** *I want to suggest to you two things: first of all, that you were keen to have a press briefing in 1998.*
>
> **Zuckerman:** *No.*
>
> **Coonan:** *Because of the history of the previous one.*
>
> **Zuckerman:** *No.*
>
> **Coonan:** *Because you thought it would reflect well, that is to say the findings in the 1998 Lancet would reflect well on the Medical School.*
>
> **Zuckerman:** *With the greatest respect, the answer to all these statements are categorically no. My position was to defend the Medical School's reputation on flawed research. Every time I went to Geneva to the World Health Organisation [WHO] I was challenged why was the Medical School, and I in particular as the Dean, as the director of the one of the [WHO] laboratories, did not challenge and stop this particular publicity which was damaging the reputation of the school. It certainly was not enhancing the reputation of the Medical School as you allege, it is the reverse. It was extremely damaging to the Medical School.*

The dean had clearly been subjected to considerable political pressure. His evidence segued into his statement that included "flawed research," which had not been relevant to the question. Coonan pressed on:

> **Coonan:** *I am sorry to have to suggest this but your recollection and reconstruction of this is inadequate and inaccurate.*

> **Zuckerman:** *I absolutely reject this. I resent the statement. I really do resent this. Mr Chairman, I absolutely object and reject this.*

In fact, Zuckerman protested to the GMC Panel chairman, Dr. Kumar, that Coonan was making statements on his behalf rather than putting a question. The chairman rejected this. In fact, Zuckerman's protest led to him being reprimanded by Kumar at which point he threatened to bring in his own legal representation.

Following a brief discussion, Coonan moved on to a different tack. The new topic was that of a video news release (VNR). As chairman of the media committee, Zuckerman had commissioned the production of a VNR for distribution to interested media outlets. This was to contain interviews with various authors of *The Lancet* paper, shots of the hospital, and an interview with the parents of an affected child who had been treated at the Royal Free. In evidence, Hutchinson recalled that in a press release approved by Zuckerman, at the bottom under "NOTES TO EDITORS," there was the statement "we have available a colour still of a child being immunized and a VNR." One might reasonably ask why the dean approved the circulation of an image of a child being vaccinated when, apparently, this thorny subject had specifically been censored by him.

A comparison of the unused material[9] and Zuckerman's testimony reflects the way in which Zuckerman's answers were refashioned over time. On August 7, 2006, a GMC lawyer from Field Fisher Waterhouse (FFW) put it to him that

> *One of our witnesses has told us that you decided that a VNR about Dr Wakefield's work should be distributed to the press prior to the press conference. Why did you think a VNR would be appropriate?*[10]

Zuckerman flatly denied being aware of any VNR. He claimed to have seen it only after the press briefing, had "completely disapproved" of it, and insisted that he had asked Hutchinson to stop any distribution of the VNR to the press.

Coonan raised the issue of the VNR at the GMC, leading Zuckerman patiently onward through a maze of contradiction and irrelevance.

> **Coonan:** *There was prepared, was there not, what was called a video news release?*

> **Zuckerman:** *I think that the issue of a video was discussed certainly and there is no question that I agreed to it.*

Having stated in August 2006 that he knew nothing of the VNR, by 2007 Zuckerman was, in contradiction, stating that there was "no question" that he had "agreed" to its production.

Coonan moved onto the VNR's content.

> **Coonan:** *Are you saying you did not know about the content of the video news release before the press conference?*

> **Zuckerman:** *No. As I say, I knew that there was going to be one after the press briefing and secondly, I also saw captions that were to be used... Having seen the sub-headings – and I amended some of them – the press officer from the hospital wrote to me to say that this did not mean that these were going to be the ultimate subheadings, because the wordings may well be changed. To my horror, in fact the wordings were changed when I saw the video after the press briefing and I instructed Mrs Hutchison not to release the video because it did not reflect either the contents of the press briefing nor did it reflect the contents of The Lancet paper, but she unfortunately told me that the actual video had been released before the press briefing, which surprised me.*

Zuckerman claimed in evidence that he was surprised by the VNR's content and that he was unaware that it had been produced by an independent company rather than the school's medical illustration department. Hutchinson, on the other hand, stated:

> *I would have expected the Dean to be aware of the various stages and to have seen a draft of the script before it was finalised. I remember that he took a close interest in the arrangements. As the VNR was funded by the medical school, I would expect that the Dean would have sanctioned the instruction of Campaign Productions and would have had to have approved the costs.*

`chinson continued:

I do not recall the Dean instructing me not to release the video... I am unable to say whether or not I discussed the minutiae with the Dean but I can say that he did show a close interest in the arrangements for the VNR, press statement and the press briefing. I do not recall the Dean being surprised at the time the VNR was produced or the press statement released. I do not recall ever being told by the Dean that he was not happy about these arrangements.

Zuckerman deviated on the point of who produced the VNR. Coonan had to put some tension on the line to get him back.

Coonan: *Let us just take stock. I am not for present purposes concerned with who produced it.*

Zuckerman: *But I am.*

Coonan: *I appreciate you might be. With respect, I am just asking the questions. If you need to mention other matters, they can be dealt with in cross-examination. Do you follow? That is the process we have. I am just seeking to establish the extent to which you were aware of the content of the video news release before the press briefing.*

Zuckerman: *I was aware of the subheadings, not the contents. Also, I was told that these were subject to alteration.*

Coonan: *Were you sent the script of the video news release before the press briefing?*

Zuckerman: *No.*

Coonan took Zuckerman to a memo from Hutchinson to him from the unused material — that is, information that the prosecution had, for obvious reasons, decided not to introduce in evidence.

Coonan: *I have asked you to look at this because when I asked you whether you had seen a copy of the script of the video news release, you said you had not.*

The memo, dated January 28, 1998, refers to the fact that a transcript of the interviews for the VNR was to be forwarded to the dean. There is a handwritten note in the date of receipt stamp that stated "discuss the 28/1 please return to Phillipa." It was initialed by Zuckerman.

Zuckerman was hauled in toward the boat — toward the keen steel of Coonan's gaff. Next came the crucial evidence relating to my position on MMR vaccine.

> **Coonan:** *Professor Zuckerman, I want to go back, please, to the preparations for the press briefing. When you were being asked about these matters by Field Fisher Waterhouse[11] in September of last year, you told them that you did not know that Dr Wakefield would suggest the use of monovalent vaccines in place of the MMR vaccine.*

> **Zuckerman:** *That is correct.*

> **Coonan:** *That is correct, is it? You did not know that?*

> **Zuckerman:** *I knew that he held that view. I knew that the press briefing was to be restricted to the pathological changes in the gut. The issue of vaccines was not relevant. I was reassured on this by Professor Pounder, I was reassured on this by Dr Wakefield, I was reassured by the letter that Professor Pounder wrote to the Chief Medical Officer on 15 January, assuring him that the press briefing would be restricted to pathological changes and therefore the issue of monovalent, polyvalent or any other vaccines was not an issue to be discussed at the press briefing, merely the pathological changes.*

Roy Pounder, my boss, had written twice to the Chief Medical Officer. Once was on January 9, 1998, offering to send him an advance copy of the paper in line with previous responsible efforts to keep his department informed. The second letter was sent, dated January 18, 1998, enclosing a draft of the paper and also alerting the CMO to the fact that some members of the team would be likely to recommend single vaccines. It indicated to him that he may wish to have enough single vaccines on hand to deal with increased demand. In neither of Pounder's letters was there even a hint of reassurance about confining the press briefing to a discussion of the bowel disease in autistic children as Zuckerman claimed. Similarly, no such discussion had ever taken place between Zuckerman and me. Coonan continued:

> **Coonan:** *Did one of the contents of the material which you were shown have Dr Wakefield, in accordance with the script, saying that the monovalent, the single vaccine, to be [sic] safer than the polyvalent vaccine?*

Zuckerman challenged Coonan to produce any document supporting this position. But Coonan held back, stretching the moment a little longer.

> **Coonan:** *I just want to ask you this. Can you remember, before the press briefing, being aware of Dr Wakefield's position on the debate between poly and monovalent?*

> **Zuckerman:** *Yes, indeed, I was and I have already said so. Let me just qualify this. It was an exchange of correspondence between Dr Wakefield and I where he wrote to me, assuring me that he had confidence in* **polyvalent**[12] *vaccines.*

So, according to Zuckerman, there was correspondence, strangely not contained in the files submitted by him to the GMC, that assured him of my confidence in MMR vaccine. Coonan took him to that correspondence with the rider "since you have raised it." Smith, senior prosecuting counsel, interjected on the basis that Zuckerman needed time to review documents that had just been "banged in front of him after 11 years." Coonan invited Zuckerman to take as much time as he needed. Zuckerman, even before he had received this evidence from the clerk stated, "I am aware of my reply, but I just need to see this letter, which was not in my file." Like an Inca priest predicting the long-range weather from entrails, he was ready with a reply to a letter that was not yet in his hand, not in his files, and one which he hadn't apparently read in 11 years. Coonan presented him with my letter to Walker-Smith — that was copied to him and stated my position on MMR — and Zuckerman's response.

> **Coonan:** *The correspondence in effect reflects, does it not – these are my words; you may disagree with them and please feel free to do so – the polarisation of view which had emerged by that stage? Is that fair? I am just seeking a form of words to summarise the two positions which we see in these two documents.*

> **Zuckerman:** *It is stating Dr Wakefield's position, yes. Absolutely.*

> **Coonan:** *In relation to the fourth paragraph in the letter to Professor Walker-Smith which was copied to you, you see the beginning of the paragraph. It says this: "In view of this, if..." My emphasis – "... my opinion is sought, I cannot support the continued use of the polyvalent MMR vaccine. I have no doubt of the value of the continued use of the* **monovalent**[12] *vaccines, and will continue to support their use until the*

case has been proven one way or another of the measles link to chronic inflammatory bowel disease."

In the course of your evidence a few minutes ago, before you took a few minutes to read the correspondence, I think you told the Panel that Dr Wakefield had assured you that he had confidence in the polyvalent vaccine. In fact, he did not, did he?

*Zuckerman: So it appears, but from the conversations I had with Dr Wakefield, he assured me on three points: that **polyvalent**[12] vaccines are useful, that his views on **monovalent**[12] vaccines, which were well-known and discussed with the press in 1997, never mind 1998, were well-known, and he assured me that the issue of vaccines will not be discussed at the press briefing.*

Zuckerman had told the GMC that he had had correspondence from me "assuring [him] that [I] had confidence in **polyvalent**[12] vaccines." There was no such correspondence. Quite the opposite; the correspondence showed that I was emphatic about my lack of confidence in MMR. Now Zuckerman was asking the panel to believe that these reassurances were contained in *conversations* between us where my position had shifted dramatically. Again, no such conversations had ever taken place. Coonan put this to Zuckerman:

Coonan: Professor Zuckerman, I have to suggest to you that that was not an assurance that he gave you in January 1998, because that is the very opposite of what that fourth paragraph is saying, is it not? "… if my opinion is sought, I cannot support the continued use of the polyvalent vaccine."

Zuckerman: I think that you should address this question of whether he discussed this with me to Dr Wakefield, who will have to answer it under oath.

Coonan: I am just going to suggest, and content myself with suggesting for present purposes, that your recollection is at fault.

Zuckerman: I have to disagree with your suggestion.

When Zuckerman was asked about his response to my letter and, in particular, his use of the word "monovalent" in the setting of "You support the continued use of the monovalent vaccines and you write that you have no doubt of their value," he claimed in the interview with FFW in 2006 and again under oath in his direct evidence to the GMC to have made a typographical error. Apparently, he had intended to use the word "polyvalent" (MMR) instead. In fact, when he wrote "monovalent" he was responding directly to the line in my letter that read "I have no doubt of the value of the continued use of the monovalent vaccines, and will continue to support their use." Zuckerman was to make the same alleged "typographical" error twice in the same letter when in the final paragraph he reiterated, "It is vital, in your own interests and that of children, that you clearly state your support for monovalent vaccination." In pressing Zuckerman on the reference to monovalent vaccines in Pounder's letter to the CMO, Zuckerman had a meltdown. In light of this, Coonan started but never got to complete his question:

> *Coonan: At any rate, knowing what was in, at the very least, this* [Wakefield's] *letter and knowing what was in the Professor Pounder correspondence which you had referred to, the correspondence with the Chief Medical Officer ---*

> *Zuckerman: No, no. I did not see that letter. The letter I saw was where he was talking about monovalent vaccines. I only saw the internet more recently. I had no knowledge of that letter. I was referring to the letter that he wrote to the Chief Medical Officer, assuring the Chief Medical Officer that nothing would be discussed other than pathological changes. That letter is on file somewhere.*

Coonan tried again, but Zuckerman, in a state of high anxiety, leapt straight in.

> *Coonan: This is a letter from Professor Pounder to ---*

> *Zuckerman: The Chief Medical Officer. The second letter I did not see until I saw it on Mr Deer's internet site.*

By now, Coonan was growing impatient of Zuckerman's dissembling.

> *Coonan: We will leave that to one side, because I am concerned with your state of mind at the time.*

> *Zuckerman: My state of mind?*

> *Coonan: Yes.*

Zuckerman: Good heavens. I find this quite offensive. What are you implying?

While Coonan was referring to what Zuckerman was *actually* thinking in 1997, Coonan's reference to his "state of mind" caused Zuckerman to lose it. His sense of affront cannot be captured on a page. Coonan pressed on:

Coonan: The fact is that, knowing what you did from this correspondence, from this exchange of letters between Dr Wakefield to Professor Walker-Smith and your reply, you did not stop the press conference.

Zuckerman: No, I did not. I should have done but I was assured that this would not arise. So, there we are.

Coonan: At the press conference, I am going to suggest to you that, at some stage, a particular journalist raised the question – and this is a summary, not a verbatim account – of what parents should do in relation to MMR and you directed the journalist to Dr Wakefield for an answer.

Zuckerman: I directed the question to Dr Wakefield for an answer, yes.

Coonan: After Dr Wakefield gave his answer, you explained to the journalists gathered there the basis of Dr Wakefield's theory, namely by which the immune system is challenged by the combination of three vaccines. That was his theory.

Zuckerman: What I recall happened is as follows. The question was asked. I certainly directed the question to Dr Wakefield for an answer. When he gave his answer, which I did not expect... The reason why I directed his question – and let me illustrate to you my state of mind at the time – was as follows. Single measles vaccines were not available in the United Kingdom, were not used in the United Kingdom, and were not used in any of the western countries, the United States or Canada. I knew that Dr Wakefield had a young family. It therefore was inevitable that they were protected with MMR and the expectation was that he would say, "Yes, I used the MMR to vaccinate my children". When he replied in the way that he did, I immediately directed the question to Dr Simon Murch, who was the paediatrician, who rejected that completely and said that he had full confidence in MMR, which I did as well. That is the position. Unless you show me the video, I really cannot remember word for word what happened, but that was the state of mind, to use your term, behind this.

In fact, the video of the press briefing was played to the GMC hearing. It bore little, if any, resemblance to Zuckerman's recollection of what he said was his "state of mind." Captured on the video was the inevitable question of what parents should do about vaccination as Zuckerman's briefing turned into a free-ranging Q&A. Zuckerman had told FFW in 2006 that my statement about splitting the MMR vaccine "had been outrageous." The truth was that Zuckerman had known for some weeks exactly what my position on MMR was. According to Hutchinson, Zuckerman had called for a press briefing precisely to reflect the differing opinions on MMR, and as she said in her witness statement, "He controlled who spoke and when." If he had had the concerns that he protested to the GMC, then he could have prevented the briefing, banned me from attending, or, at the very least, directed the question to someone else who continued to support MMR. He did none of these things. He asked me to respond to the journalist's question. I did so exactly in accordance with my stated beliefs and intentions.

Before the GMC, Zuckerman expressed the surprise that he had felt because "single vaccines were not available in the UK"; wrong, they were. Zuckerman had no basis for believing that my children had received the MMR vaccine. And he certainly did not, as he said, "immediately direct the question to Simon Murch." Instead, with the calm authority of a man who had previously described himself to the GMC lawyers as "the world's leading virologist in clinical virology,"[13] he delivered a prepared explanation of a plausible basis for my concerns.

In fact, at the press briefing, Zuckerman had stated:

> *Can I just try and actually answer that question more precisely? MMR consists of 3 live attenuated virus strains. In other words we are administering to the children in the MMR three attenuated vaccine strains against measles, against mumps, against rubella. A combination of three different viruses… it is theoretically possible that the immune system would be challenged by 3 separate viruses and that would be the rationale I think for Dr Wakefield's recommendation for giving these vaccines separately and of course before the MMR was introduced these preparations were available as monovalent vaccines."* [Remainder of recording inaudible.]

After a brief interruption from the floor and a statement about how safe vaccines were, he continued:

> One possible explanation is that at the age of one the immune system is not fully developed. Therefore by challenging it with three live viral, live attenuated strains may be associated with side effects.

He had provided support for my position! It was only later that he asked Murch for his opinion. Rather than Zuckerman's portrayal to the GMC of Murch's words said to "reject... completely" the idea that MMR may be linked with this new syndrome, Murch had actually endorsed the possibility that, for reasons of a poorly functioning immune system, some children "may have difficulty in handling viruses."

In reviewing the video of the press briefing, it was evident that Zuckerman was referring in his commentary to pre-prepared notes. Having previously told the GMC that vaccines were not to be discussed, it seemed curious that his notes at the press briefing likely included this very topic.

There can be little doubt that the GMC Panel might have been persuaded that, in me, they were dealing with a true villain based upon my ex-dean's damning indictment. If so, they were misled.

The GMC's lawyers had briefed Zuckerman in advance of his oral testimony, warning him not to be caught off guard by hostile allegations that he had "purposefully directed a question to Dr Wakefield at the press conference, knowing what his answer would be i.e. that it would be controversial."[14] Zuckerman described this as "a lie," but that he could respond to it. The evidence would suggest otherwise.

Zuckerman was a man of conflicting agendas; on the one hand, his role as dean had been to support academic freedom. On the other, he was put under considerable political pressure from the Department of Health and World Health Organization (WHO) in respect of my legitimate research into vaccine safety (see endnotes 2, 3, 5, and 7 of Chapter 3, "The Dean's Dilemma" and endnote 8 of this chapter). While initially using the autism work to promote the medical school in the media, it rapidly became a decaying albatross about his neck. In a rather clumsy volte face before the GMC hearing, Zuckerman's imperfect memory was exposed. Time and again, he was undone by the contradictions between his testimony, the documented facts, and the opinions of other witnesses. In the end, he did protest too much.

Endnotes

[1] January 12, 1998 letter from AJW to John Walker-Smith, copied to Professor Arie Zuckerman, Professor Roy Pounder, Dr. Simon Murch, Dr. Mike Thomson, and Dr. Mark Berelowitz.

[2] Intestinal disease.

[3] Emphasis added.

[4] Single vaccines; emphasis added.

[5] IBD – inflammatory bowel disease.

[6] Names removed for legal reasons.

[7] Emphasis added.

[8] Witness statement of Phillipa Hutchinson for Field Fisher Waterhouse. September 18, 2006.

[9] Information that the prosecution decided not to introduce in evidence.

[10] Attendance note from GMC lawyers. August 7, 2006. Questions pages 2 and 3; answers page 3.

[11] GMC lawyers.

[12] Emphasis added.

[13] Attendance note: Quote from Zuckerman to GMC lawyers in GMC "unused material." August 7, 2006

[14] Attendance note: Quote from Zuckerman to GMC lawyers in GMC "unused material." May 16, 2006. Para 6.

CHAPTER SEVEN

Horton and *The Lancet*

Texas, February 29, 2008: The filing cabinet's top drawer was crammed and fully open, threatening to topple. Carmel, my long-suffering wife, was oblivious, her mind elsewhere. Shipping the Wakefields' worldly goods from Kew Gardens, London, to professional and political exile in Texas had not been without problems. Two filing cabinets had remained in a warehouse in London's Docklands and only threat of litigation had secured their onward passage to the US. And the documents they held were to be key in the unfolding mystery. Our longitudes were now reversed: she was in Texas and I was in London preparing to take the witness stand before the GMC's Fitness to Practise Panel. "I've found it!" she exclaimed over the phone, "I've found the original 'Rouse letter.'"

So much of the misrepresentation of the work of my colleagues and me has been centered on attempts to discredit it, starting with the allegation of a "hidden conflict of interest." This was triggered by Brian Deer's false assertion that *The Lancet* 1998 study had been funded by the UK's Legal Aid Board and that this "fact" had been kept secret from both *The Lancet* and my colleagues. In my opinion, leading the disorderly vanguard of those seeking to distance themselves from *The Lancet* paper in 2004, has been the editor Richard Horton.

Richard Horton has been editor of *The Lancet* since 1995. As editor, he has overall responsibility for *everything* that is published in the journal. Following submission of "That Paper" to *The Lancet* in mid-1997,[1] Horton and his team had sent it out to four independent and anonymous reviewers. The paper was published in February 1998 with an accompanying editorial from the US Centers for Disease Control and Prevention (CDC), warning gravely of the dangers of measles. Subsequent exchanges in the "Correspondence" columns of *The Lancet* were charged as would be expected. One correspondent was Dr. A. Rouse, a public health doctor from the west of England. His letter was published on May 2, 1998. As published – and this is crucial – it read:

After reading Andrew Wakefield and colleagues' article I did a simple internet search and found the Society for Autistically Handicapped. I downloaded a 48 page fact sheet produced for the society by Dawbarns a firm of solicitors in King's Lynn. It seems likely that some of the children investigated by Wakefield et al came to attention because of the activities of this society and information from the parents referred in this way would suffer from recall bias. It is a pity that Wakefield et al do not identify the manner in which the 12 children were referred (e.g. from local GPs, self referral via parents or secondary/ tertiary or international referral). Furthermore if some children were referred directly or indirectly because of the activities of the Society for the Autistically Handicapped, Wakefield should have declared his cooperation with that organization.

It is uncertain as to how much attention Rouse had actually paid to *The Lancet* paper itself since, in relation to patient referral, the paper stated quite clearly that the children were "self-referred," meaning that the parents had initiated the request to be seen at the Royal Free. The paper also described the mode of referral via the child's doctor.

While I had never heard of the Society for the Autistically Handicapped, my role in the litigation was no secret, having been reported in the national press as early as November 1996.[2] I duly responded to the various issues raised by the correspondents. John Walker-Smith and Simon Murch, anxious for personal reasons not to be associated with vaccine litigation, approved my response but chose to keep their distance. My response to the Rouse letter read:

A. Rouse suggests that litigation bias might exist by virtue of information that he has downloaded from the internet from the Society of the Autistically Handicapped.

Pausing there, it would be reasonable to ask why I would refer to "litigation bias." It is a most unusual term and certainly not included in Rouse's letter as eventually published in *The Lancet*. Suffice it to say that I was reminded of its actual content 10 years later following Carmel's discovery.

Continuing with my response to *The Lancet* in 1998, I went on to describe my past and continuing involvement in the MMR litigation:

Only one author (AJW) has agreed to help evaluate a small number of these children on behalf of the Legal Aid Board. These children have all been seen expressly on the basis that they were referred through the normal channels (e.g. from GPs, child psychiatrist or community paediatricians) on the merit of their symptoms. AJW had never heard of the Society for the Autistically Handicapped and no fact sheet has been provided for them to distribute to interested parties. The only fact sheet that we have produced is for GPs which describes the background and protocol for investigation of children with autism and gastrointestinal symptoms. Finally all those children referred to us (including 53 who have already been investigated and those on a waiting list that extends into 1999) have come through the formal channels described above. No conflict of interest exists.

That was where matters rested in 1998 and, given that my involvement with the lawyers seeking to establish whether there was a case in law against the vaccine manufacturers had been widely reported in the lay press and now confirmed in this exchange of letters in *The Lancet*, as far as I was concerned, there it would rest. Clearly at the time, Horton did not feel it necessary to explore this matter further.

In the event, as time moved on, the cauldron of litigation, claim, and counter-claim came to the boil, and by the end of 2001, my career in Britain was over. Over the intervening years there have been further publications, some in *The Lancet*[8] that have been used to support claims that any links between MMR vaccine and autism have been disproved. These publications have often been heralded by a fanfare of publicity and Horton's appearance in the media seeking to exonerate the MMR vaccine (see below) from any possible link with autism.

Horton had been under considerable pressure since the publication of "That Paper." He wrote a book in 2003 titled *Second Opinion*. The MMR issue is described. Horton rehearses what a terrible time he had following publication of *The Lancet* paper in 1998; how he was telephoned by the former president of the UK's Academy of Medical Sciences "in a fury about the publication of a paper that raised questions about MMR." He tells of a dreadful experience at a dinner party where he was asked if he would ever be forgiven for this publication and its effects. We agonize with him as he relives the process of sending the paper for four independent reviews prior to accepting it, the editing to ensure that the readers knew there was no proof that MMR vaccine caused "this new syndrome," how the preliminary nature of the findings was emphasized, and how the public was reinformed of the importance of measles vaccination. He shares with us the sometimes "highly personal" attacks on him — "unusual in scientific debate." Finally, Horton confesses that, with regard to the public's concern about the safety of the vaccine, "despite our best efforts as editors a snowballing effect happened."

The drama intensifies as Horton's readers are told how my recommendation in Feburary 1998 that parents might opt for single vaccines until the issue had been resolved scientifically was

> ...*for all practical purposes a recommendation to parents not to have their children vaccinated at all since the components were not available separately in the U.K.*

This is a serious allegation and it is false; single vaccines *were* licensed and available at the time. I knew this when making my recommendation; otherwise I would not have made it. The importation license for the single vaccines was withdrawn by the Department of Health in August 1998, meaning choice was no longer available via the National Health Service.[3] At a time when demand was greatest, the option for concerned parents had been removed, effectively putting protection of MMR vaccination policy before protection of children.

Horton tells readers how "embarrassingly naïve" his actions were in 1998, how he should have tried to persuade me not to have recommended splitting the vaccine, how he was too "laissez-faire," and how he failed to manage the media at that time but has learned now how integral this is to his responsibilities. But his book also tells us that he does not regret publishing the original paper since progress in medicine depends on the "free expression of new ideas," and in science it was only this commitment to free expression which "shook free the tight grip of religion on the way humans understood their world." My work, he suggests, has opened up an important new field of science — the relationship between the brain and the intestine in autism. He goes on to tell those still awake that I have published extensively about the risks of MMR and measles infection since 1998, but that others have

> ...*convincingly refuted any association between the vaccine and autism in large studies across different populations... Not one person or group has confirmed the original findings in the Lancet paper.*

This is the mantra, the hungry falsehood, handed down to the media by the DoH, swallowed, and regurgitated in the popular press on a regular basis. With respect to my colleagues, Horton goes on to say that John Walker-Smith

...was and remains sceptical of a direct link with the MMR vaccine but believes that there appears to be a small highly selected group of children where there is a risk.

Horton's 2003 book concludes with the lessons to be learned from this "sad affair" that

...has left Wakefield's reputation unfairly in tatters, virtually unemployable in the UK for the work he wanted to do.

Meanwhile, as Christmas approached, Brian Deer the freelance journalist, unknown to all but a few, was thumbing through documents provided to him in the most extraordinary circumstances. Strictly confidential medical records of disabled children had been provided to him apparently by the North London Special Health Authority that had oversight for the Royal Free.

On the Monday morning of February 9, 2004, Carmel, alone in the UK with our four children, lost her job as medicolegal consultant to Stoke Mandeville Hospital due to regulatory changes. In the school yard, one of her friends tried to cheer her up: "Well at least things can't get any worse!" On her return home, she received a call from Abel Hadden, a public relations consultant, informing her that Deer was seeking a response to various allegations about me and that he was about to go public with these allegations. The nub of them was that I had published research in *The Lancet* in 1998, and that I had been paid £55,000.00 by the Legal Aid Board to do this, despite the fact that the clinical investigations described in the paper had been paid for by the National Health Service. Deer also alleged that none of my colleagues at the Royal Free knew that I was helping investigate a potential claim on behalf of autistic children and that I had plotted with lawyer Richard Barr. Together, according to Deer, we had contrived an MMR problem in order to sue the vaccine manufacturers. Additionally, it was Deer's "clinical" opinion that the tests on these children were inappropriate, invasive, and unethical.

Meanwhile, Deer had telephoned Horton to whet his appetite and propose a full face-to-face expose of my wickedness. Horton's response was described by Deer in an e-mail to his commissioning editor, Paul Nukki, as enthusiastic saying, "if this holds up in terms of documentation, this could be grounds to retract the paper."[5] Strangely prescient words it would seem, as I am writing this 6 years later when Horton has done that very thing.

I flew back from the US and walked into a meeting with representatives of *The Sunday Times* while Deer tantalized Horton and colleagues with a 3-hour presentation that revealed the fruits of his labors – "evidence" of my alleged financial and ethical impropriety.

That same afternoon a meeting was hastily arranged at *The Lancet's* offices between the senior authors of the paper. I had not seen Walker-Smith, Murch, or Horton for many years. Unfortunately, both of my colleagues had given interviews to Deer in the meantime that led him to believe that they had had no knowledge of my involvement in the Legal Aid Board work. While this misunderstanding may have arisen out of the manner of Deer's questioning, it had the effect of facilitating what was to become the longest GMC inquiry in history.

Horton's precise understanding of what Deer had alleged is important because it is inconsistent with what he was to claim later on. Horton set out his understanding of the allegations. It was clear that he was operating on the basis of the allegation that *The Lancet* report had been funded by the LAB and that this obvious conflict of interest had not been disclosed. Paraphrasing here, Horton opened with the allegations to the effect that: I've had a reporter from *The Sunday Times* here with a Liberal Democrat MP by the name of Evan Harris. The journalist – Deer was his name – alleged that you Andy [we were on first name terms at this stage] were given £55,000 by lawyers to investigate some of *The Lancet* children, that the work reported in *The Lancet* was funded by lawyers and this fact was not declared to me or disclosed in the paper, and that you kept this secret from your coauthors.

Apparently, Murch's "jaw dropped." I responded that, in fact, *The Lancet* paper was not funded by the LAB or by lawyers – that the funding was for an entirely separate scientific study looking for evidence of measles virus in the diseased intestine of affected children. The children were all referred for clinical investigation of their symptoms, and their referral, which predated any legal involvement, had nothing to do with lawyers or litigation. I stated that, in my opinion – effectively the test of conflict of interest required of an author by *The Lancet* at that time – there was no conflict of interest. Presented with this apparently new take on the matter, Horton paused and proposed, with a renewed sense of purpose, that there was "the possibility of a *perceived* conflict of interest." I was perplexed and, as Horton was later to confirm in response to the panel chairman's question at the GMC, "surprised." The possible perceptions of others were not part of *The Lancet's* disclosure requirements in 1996-98. The children had not been litigants at the time they were referred to Walker-Smith, their clinical investigation was not influenced by whether they might litigate at some future time, and I — the only member of the Royal Free team to be involved in litigation — played no active part in the interpretation of clinical findings in these children. My contribution, in addition to the original ideas, had been the collation of the data and drafting of the paper based upon the findings of others. Horton and I were to argue back and forth on the definition of a conflict for much of the rest of the meeting; it finished with us completely at odds on this issue.

Further allegations from Deer hit closer to home for Walker-Smith and Murch. The accusation that children had been "sourced" by lawyers rather than being clinical referrals from other doctors and the claim that the children had been subjected to invasive procedures as an experiment were deeply disturbing.

Horton gave the three of us 48 hours to piece together events that had taken place up to 8 years earlier and to come back to him with our written statements in order that these could be published in *The Lancet* online that Friday. Assignments given, the meeting in Horton's office broke up. What remained was a sense of despair — real despair. One thing that I was to recollect much later was that on Horton's desk that day, untouched and unread during the course of our meeting, was a copy of the letters page of *The Lancet* – none other than the Rouse letter and my response from May 2, 1998.

For our assignments, I was to deal with issues of litigation and conflict of interest; Walker-Smith was to deal with the clinical referral and investigation that had taken place; Murch was to address the issue of ethical approval and Professor Hodgson, the clinical dean, with the medical school's position. There was an urgent meeting of the latter three, accompanied by Horton, at the Royal Free the next day to review the clinical records, departmental logs of admissions, and procedures and ethics committee applications and approvals. I was not invited. Following my forced departure from the Royal Free, many documents had been necessarily destroyed either for reasons of confidentiality or simply weight of numbers. What remained had been gathering dust in random piles in my garage. Had the real Rouse letter come to light at that time, the story might have been a very different one.

On the last day of the children's half-term break, Friday, February 20, Carmel took the two youngest children, Imogen and Corin, to see *School of Rock.* In the middle of it, I called on her cell phone with the news that I had just had a telephone call from Horton who had told me how much respect he had for me, how he did not doubt my honesty and integrity, and how he sympathized with the invidious position in which I found myself. He professed to be full of admiration for the fact that I had been able to put up with so much adversity for so long. She was silent. "What the hell is he up to?" was her terse response. Only then did I realize that Horton's call heralded a new turn of events — and that nothing good would come of it.

Within hours of this call, Horton was on every major news channel proclaiming that *The Lancet* paper of 1998 should never have been published. He declared the paper to be "fatally flawed." He told the BBC: "…if we had known the conflict of interest Dr Wakefield had in this work I think that would have strongly affected the peer reviewers about the credibility of this work and in my judgment it would have been rejected."

Much later I learned, via a friend of one of the deputy editors of *The Sunday Times*, that it was Horton going public in this way that led to the paper's decision to publish Deer's article. Horton had created a media monster thirsty for my blood, and despite anxieties about the article's factual basis, the editorial team at *The Sunday Times* decided to run it.

Horton appeared the following morning on the *Today* program (the UK's flagship radio news program) with John Humphreys, the elder statesman of British media inquisitors. Horton told listeners that it was his view that the work was *entirely* flawed. Pressed on this by Humphreys, he was forced to agree that the finding of a new syndrome of autism and bowel disease was not flawed, rather it needed to be investigated further. When questioned about MMR, the seasoned skeptic in Humphreys was surprised as Horton declared that it was "absolutely safe."

I was headline news in the next day's edition of *The Sunday Times* on February 22. By Monday, my detractors were rushing to give sound bites after *The Sunday Times* article. Professor Liam Donaldson, the Chief Medical Officer, took his opportunity on the *Today* program when he observed:

> *Now a darker side of this work has shown through, with the ethical conduct of the research and this is something that has to be looked at.*

Meanwhile, on Independent Television news, Prime Minister Tony Blair (who had been so secretive about the fact that his son Leo had not had the MMR) remarked, "I hope now that people see the situation is somewhat different from what they were led to believe."

Elsewhere, Deer was busy preparing an indignant, public-spirited complaint to the GMC alleging "possible professional misconduct of Andrew Wakefield and his colleagues Walker-Smith and Murch." Also vocal after *The Sunday Times* article were Shadow Health Minister[4] Dr. Liam Fox and, once again, the Chief Medical Officer, Dr. Liam Donaldson. Both called for an enquiry by the GMC. Ironically, I had beaten them all to it. I had already called on the GMC for an investigation of the matter myself.

It was another journalist, Jeremy Laurence, health correspondent for *The Independent*, who first jogged my memory when he wrote in his paper later that week to say that my involvement in the litigation was not hidden, but had been disclosed in *The Lancet* a few weeks following publication. As a result of this revelation I sought an apology from Horton through lawyers Messrs. Carter-Ruck.

> *We have been consulted by our client, Dr Andrew Wakefield with regard to the statement which you issued on the 20th February which together with interviews you have given, has received widespread media attention, as was only to be expected.*
>
> *Our client, as you will know, entirely rejects your assertion that his work for the Legal Aid Board gave rise to a conflict of interest in relation to the paper published in The Lancet in February 1998, let alone that it left our client's work "fatally flawed" as you have alleged. This, however, is a matter which our client considers may be best resolved through a GMC enquiry, which has been proposed and which our client welcomes.*
>
> *There can, however, be no dispute concerning our client's good faith. The plain implications of the statement you have made is that our client, for nearly six years, withheld not only from The Lancet but from his colleagues that he was also engaged by the Legal Aid Board to conduct research. This, as you know, is not true. There was no secret and our client made no secret of his work for the Legal Aid Board. Indeed, the letter published by our client in the Lancet on 2 May 1998 makes crystal clear not only that the fact that our client was engaged in other research was publicly available on the internet but also that*

the very issue of an alleged conflict was raised and refuted by our client at the time, in a letter which, as Editor, you were responsible for passing for publication in the Lancet. It is in these circumstances a matter of grave concern, that, six years after all of the relevant facts were in your knowledge, you chose not only to dismiss our client's work but to cast doubt on his honesty.

The purpose of this letter, whilst reserving all our client's legal rights, is to invite you to agree promptly to publish a full apology to our client, in a form, manner, and terms to be agreed by him. We trust we shall hear from you within seven days.

Needless to say, we never received an apology and were not in a position financially to take the matter further. Appealing to Horton's sense of fair play had been naïve. His response through Olswang, *The Lancet's* law firm, is important and is referred to later.

Horton, however, clearly remained troubled that he had not done enough. As he had indicated to Deer when the allegations were first made, he might have grounds to retract the paper – expunge it from history. In the event, all that he could manage was a "partial retraction," i.e., that any interpretation of a possible association between the children's condition and MMR vaccination was in error. His idea, offered to me over the telephone as an olive branch, was ludicrous on at least two counts. First, the 1998 paper had never provided the interpretation that MMR caused autism; second, it is impossible to retract a possibility. I considered that such a retraction would be deeply insulting to the parents of the children involved, rendering their story somehow invalid, in the absence of appropriate investigation. Ten of the thirteen authors, some of whom had listened firsthand to the parents' stories and with good reason believed them, were persuaded to join the partial retraction of an interpretation. This letter of "retraction of an association" was published on March 6, 2004, which was 16 days after the matter had first been raised. The message inevitably conveyed in the media was that the entire paper had been retracted and was effectively discredited.

Three of the authors, Dr. Peter Harvey, Dr. John Linnell, and I, wrote a long and detailed letter to *The Lancet* outlining why we considered any retraction to be a mockery. We explained why there was no conflict of interest and why, in the absence of a causal interpretation attributable to the MMR in *The Lancet* paper, there was nothing to withdraw. This measured and detailed letter, written by the three dissenters, was sent to *The Lancet* at the same time as the retraction letter. In the interests of fairness, both positions should and could have been viewed together. But while the retraction letter was published to a blaze of publicity, it took a further 6 weeks for our response to appear on April 17, 2004. When it did finally appear it was inserted discreetly halfway down the letter's page.

Horton's determination to wash his hands of his part in the publication of *The Lancet* paper was paying off. This was evidenced in an exchange between Member of Parliament Evan Harris (Liberal Democrat) and Crispin Davis, Chairman of Reed-Elsevier, *The Lancet's* proprietor and Horton's boss, which took place at the UK government's Science and Technology Committee on March 1, 2004. Referring to the Rouse/Wakefield exchange, Davis told Harris:

> *You can imagine that it is virtually impossible for every editor to research every single author in terms of conflict of interest, and in this one Dr Wakefield said there was no conflict of interest, and in fact three months later in written form repeated that there was no conflict of interest. In all fairness, I do not hold our editor to blame.*

As an aside, readers may be interested to know that on July 1, 2003,[9] Crispin Davis was made a non-executive director of Glaxo SmithKline, one of the largest pharmaceutical companies in the world, manufacturers of MMR, and one of the codefendants in the MMR litigation with which I was assisting the LAB. In the summer of 2004, Davis was knighted for his services to the information industry.[10]

Horton was to publish yet another book on his MMR experience, charting the events from February 22 through August 1, 2004. It was in the shops by the autumn, and he was promoting it with a lecture tour. The news of this literary event, together with further press coverage of the MMR issue, acted as a catalyst for Carmel to make contact with Horton in order to put the record straight but to little avail. On Friday, September 10, 2004, Dr. Liam Smeeth appeared on television, trumpeting his study that purported to show no link between MMR and autism. This deeply flawed paper,[6] that was conducted in a manner contrary to the authors' intentions, was proclaimed by many as the "definitive work" and the "largest study, which confirmed that there was no basis for any concerns about the link between MMR and autism." Horton was hot on his heels. He appeared on *Channel 5 News* on Friday, September 9, 2004, lauding the Smeeth paper, dismissing my work as "smoke and mirrors," reassuring the masses with the anecdote of his daughter's vaccination, and commenting on the radio poll of its listeners. The presenter may have been persuaded, but not the public.

PRESENTER: *Well that personal testimony is a very convincing argument. Let me tell you about our 5 News Club poll today. We're asking people if they're convinced the MMR vaccine is safe. 17% — Yes convinced it's safe; 83% — No not convinced it's safe.*

Horton, uncertain how the public might ever be persuaded of MMR's safety, considered this to be a disaster. He continued:

And contrary to what Dr Wakefield says, his evidence, his so-called evidence, that the measles virus is actually linked to this syndrome, you can actually find the measles virus in these children, has been refuted time and again in other investigations.

This was an interesting assertion when, at this stage, no other investigations had been reported on the detection of measles virus in the intestine of autistic children. The presenter explored Horton's position further:

"Do you think there will be any surveys, any research done, that will satisfy Dr Wakefield that his original thesis may have been mistaken?" Horton replied, *"No I don't think he will ever be satisfied. He's invested his entire career and reputation in this belief, this hypothesis. For him to refute it now would almost be a negation of his entire personality..."*

Carmel, frustrated with Horton's treatment of me, e-mailed him, threatening to go to one of his lectures to take notes for a book she was considering writing. He replied by return e-mail:[11]

You may know that I too have just finished a book, which is about to be published – called MMR: Science and Fiction. *Obviously Andrew makes repeated appearances in what I have to say, and I have tried very hard to be as balanced as I can ...I do try to write honestly about Andrew's role in this whole affair. One thing I do strongly endorse is the need to keep these debates within the community of science and medicine and not to punish, censor, or banish individuals who dissent from orthodoxy. The trick is finding the best way of doing this. I am told that Brian Deer is now making a film. His role is far from clear to me. But I do know that he is dangerous...*

Only a few days after this message, Horton wrote again about me in the British press (rather than in the "community of science and medicine" that he had mentioned):

> The career assassination of Wakefield cleansed science of an unwise agent provocateur.

In Horton's book *MMR Science and Fiction*, it may have been therapeutic for him to describe his "tight coil of suppressed frustration" after Deer's allegations and how it "was unwinding in me having been pressed into a position of extraordinary tension during the preceding six years."[7] Horton recounts for the reader how he was able to help the GMC in deciding my professional fate – help which may have assisted in this unwinding process:

> In truth they had not a clue where to begin. At a dinner I attended on 23 February, one medical regulator and I discussed the Wakefield case. He seemed unsure of how the Council could play a useful part in resolving any confusion. As we talked over coffee while the other dinner guests were departing, he scribbled down some possible lines of investigation and passed me his card, suggesting that I contact him directly if anything else came to mind. He seemed keen to pursue Wakefield, especially given ministerial interest. Here was professionally led regulation of doctors in action – notes exchanged over liqueurs in a beautifully wood-panelled room of one of medicine's most venerable institutions.

Horton advised the GMC on the way to bring me to heel. This was to be the perfect follow-through, with Horton as one of the key prosecution witnesses at the trial.

Horton also sounded a warning of the potential consequences for the prosecutors, should they fail to get a guilty verdict on their terms. There are many soundbites from him, but one in particular bears scrutiny. In April 2006, he wrote a long piece in the UK's *Guardian* newspaper. His opening paragraph read:

> It's hard to imagine that anything useful could still be written about the MMR vaccine. Too much has probably been said already, most of it either wilful nonsense or wild speculation. So I hesitate. And especially because it was I who was responsible for <u>publishing</u> – to the eternal damnation of many of my medical and public-health colleagues

– Andrew Wakefield's 1998 paper that fuelled a smouldering underground movement against the vaccine. A campaign that we now know was partly linked to efforts to win a legal claim against vaccine manufacturers.

When Wakefield walks into the GMC, he will have a national stage that has been denied him ever since he used a press conference to call for the provision of single vaccines. The outcome of the GMC's proceedings could be lose-lose for the Department of Health. For Wakefield's supporters, he will either be vindicated as a hero or go down as a martyr to his cause.

Horton is wrong: there is a great deal more to be written about MMR vaccine. And although he may not wish it, there is more to be written about Horton's own role in this affair. And it starts with the discovery of the original Rouse letter.

Endnotes

[1] GMC vs Wakefield, Walker-Smith, and Murch. Statement of Dr John Bignall (deceased), deputy editor *The Lancet*. September 13, 2005. Page 1, paras 2-4. See also: Wakefield to Else, Letter. July 3, 1997.

[2] Langdon-Down G. (1996, November 27). "Law: A shot in the Dark." *The Independent*. Page 25.

[3] Yazbak FE. The MMR and Single Measles, Mumps and Rubella Vaccines: The REAL Facts. Retrieved from http://bmj.bmjjournals.com/cgi/eletters/329/7477/1293#92190.

Buncombe A. (1998, September 1). Measles jab withdrawn due to 'high demand'. The Independent. Retrieved from http://www.independent.co.uk/news/measles-jab-withdrawn-due-to-high-demand-1195247.html

[4] Shadow Health Minister – the minority party's Health Minister.

[5] Deer to Nukki at *The Sunday Times*. E-mail. February 17, 2004.

[6] Dr. Carol M Stott BSc PhD (Cantab) CPsychol on Smeeth et al.:

Smeeth L, Cook C, Fombonne E, Heavey L, Rodrigues L, Smith P, Hall A. MMR vaccination and pervasive developmental disorders: a case-control study. *Lancet* 2004; 364:963-969 is a case-control study purportedly designed to investigate a putative association between MMR vaccination and increased risk of pervasive developmental disorders (PDD). However, problems in study design operate against the probability of detecting an increase in risk. Furthermore, there are significant changes from the methodology first proposed 2 and subsequently cited in the present paper.

The basis of a case-control study of this kind is that if the hypothesis of the putative association has any validity, one should find a difference (i.e., an "effect") between cases and controls in the proportions exposed to the vaccine.

While it is frequently acknowledged that the "effect size" is likely to be small, the consistent error is in the assumption that this derives from a small risk conferred by MMR to many individuals rather than a substantial risk to a small number of individuals with a subsequent and specific presentation. In the former situation, case-samples could appropriately be increased by adding general PDD cases, while in the latter, case groups should be limited to, and only increased by, the addition of children in the subgroup of interest. It was obviously crucial for the reported study that case groups comprised only those children presenting with regressive or late-onset PDD. Smeeth et al. state explicitly (on page 967) that they were not able to do this.

Sample size is also an issue for this study. Conditional logistic regression (clogit) was used appropriately for the matched-pair (case-control) design. Crucially, however, the only pairs contributing to such an analysis are those in which exposure differs across the pairings. Where level of exposure in the general population is high, a substantial number of case-control pairs would share the same exposure status and, thus, be excluded. Adequate study power is only maintained, therefore, by ascertaining samples large enough to allow sufficient pairs to remain. An appropriate sample size for a matched-pair design[3] with an estimated control exposure rate of 80%, a p-value of 0.05, an case-control ratio of 1:3, a correlation coefficient for case-control paired exposure of 0.8, an odds ratio (OR) of 1.2 and a power of 0.8, would be 7,145 cases. In other words, to have a 80-20 chance of observing an OR of 1.2, almost 6 times as many cases would be needed as were used in the Smeeth, et al. study. As the case group was likely to consist of only 20-50% of the relevant phenotype, the required sample size for cases rises substantially beyond this.

Finally, the study is likely to be confounded by factors affecting underlying risk of exposure between the groups. Children at higher genetic risk of disorder may remain unexposed as may children with early onset developmental difficulties. This would result in differential exposure risk between the two groups systematically acting in favor of risk of exposure in cases being lower than in controls.

References

1. Smeeth L, Cook C, Fombonne E, Heavey L, Rodrigues L, Smith P, Hall A. MMR vaccination and pervasive developmental disorders: a case-control study. *Lancet* 2004; 364: 963-969.

2. Smeeth L, Hall A, Fombonne E, Rodrigues L, Huang X, Smith P. A case-control study of autism and mumps-measles-rubella vaccination using the general practice research database: design and methodology. *BMC Public Health.* (2001) 1:2.

3. Dupont, WD. Power calculations for matched case-control studies. *Biometrics.* 1988;44:1157-1168.

[7] Horton, R. *MMR Science and Fiction.* London: Granta Books, 2004.

[8] Taylor B, Miller E, Farrington C, Petropoulous M, Favot-Mayaud I, Li J, Waight P. Autism and measles, mumps, and rubella vaccine: no epidemiological evidence for a causal association. *The Lancet.* 1999;353;2026-2029.

[9] http://uk.reuters.com/business/quotes/officerProfile?symbol=GSK.L&officerId=475638

[10] http://www.gsk.com/about/bio-davis.htm

[11] E-mails will be posted. See www.callous-regard.com.

CHAPTER EIGHT

Horton's Evidence

On Thursday, August 7, 2007, Richard Horton walked into the chamber of the GMC, affirmed that he would tell the truth and the whole truth, and began his evidence. His wife sat behind him in the public gallery. Over 2 days of oral testimony, Ms. Smith, Senior Prosecuting Counsel, appeared to be justifiably delighted with her witness as she took him through his evidence-in-chief. It is not necessary to revisit the whole of Horton's evidence, simply to deal with the part that dealt with the Rouse letter and his state of mind in 1997 and beyond.

Smith: I want to ask you about one particular letter on page 924 from someone called A. Rouse from the Department of Public Health Medicine, Wiltshire Health Authority. At this stage I want to take you to that [response] from Wakefield. I want to take you to the middle section which begins:

"A Rouse suggests that litigation bias might exist by virtue of information that he has downloaded from the internet from the Society for the Autistically Handicapped. Only one author (AJW)... has agreed to help evaluate a small number of these children on behalf of the Legal Aid Board. These children have all been seen expressly on the basis that they were referred through the normal channels (e.g. from GP, child psychiatrist or community paediatrician) on the merits of their symptoms. AJW had never heard of the Society for the Autistically Handicapped and no fact sheet has been provided for them to distribute to interested parties. The only fact sheet that we have produced is for GPs which describes the background and protocol for investigation of children with autism and gastrointestinal symptoms. Finally, all those children referred to us (including the 53 who have been investigated already, and those on the waiting list that extended into 1999) have come through the formal channels described above. No conflict of interest exists."

Smith: When you read that letter, what did you understand Dr Wakefield to mean when he said one author has agreed to help evaluate a small number of these children on behalf of the Legal Aid Board?

Horton's reply was essentially a reiteration of Olswang's earlier response to the letter from lawyers Carter-Ruck (see Chapter 7, "Horton and *The Lancet*") with some key additions.

*Horton: When I read that letter two statements stood out: first, the assertion that you concluded that paragraph with, "no conflict of interest exists". At the time, in May 1998, I had no reason, no evidence before me, to suggest that that was an untrue statement so I took that statement on trust. With respect to the sentence that you ask about specifically, "has agreed to help evaluate", I must admit I read that as something that **happened after publication. To my knowledge in February 1998 and during the peer review process going back into 1997, I was completely unaware of any potential litigation surrounding the MMR vaccine. I was not aware of the involvement of a firm of solicitors Dawbarns. I certainly was not aware of any activity going on with the Society for the Autistically Handicapped prior to the 1998 paper. I was not aware of any other relationship between Dr Wakefield and Dawbarns and Richard Barr. When I read those statements I saw this as something that was triggered by the paper rather than the paper being in some senses a culmination of events up to February 1998.**[1]*

*Smith: Looking at the wording of the sentence you referred to "only one author **has**[1] agreed to evaluate a small number of these children on behalf of the Legal Aid Board", you say you took that to mean **since the publication of the paper**[1] and we are now some three or four months on from publication of the paper.*

Horton: Yes.

Smith: Was there anything in particular about that wording which led you to think that?

*Horton: It is the **"has"** agreed. I know these are fine distinctions. If it had said "had agreed" then I would have thought that was more in the past tense. Reading "has agreed" in combination with the firm* *assertion that no conflict of interest exists, my suspicions were not raised at that time.*

Smith: *Did you accept that letter on its face value?*

Horton: *We certainly did, yes.*

"Has" and "Had"

The English usage in my letter in response to Rouse was deliberate, grammatically correct, and factually accurate. "One of the authors has agreed" is in the *present perfect* tense. The tense is used to emphasize that something not only *happened* but is *still true*. This was the case for my involvement with the legal action at the time of writing my response to Dr. Rouse in 1998.

The matter of the tense is not, as Horton has stated, a "fine distinction" but conveys, in this matter, a crucial difference in meaning that, somewhat curiously, was lost on the editor-in-chief of a major medical journal. *"Had agreed"* is the *past perfect* tense; its use would have been neither grammatically correct nor factually accurate. The use of this tense is to emphasize that something *happened* but is *not true anymore*. This was not the case at the time that I wrote to *The Lancet* in response to Rouse.

Let us examine Horton's position more closely in light of his critical misunderstanding of English grammar. First is the response, via his lawyers, to the 2004 letter seeking an apology from my lawyers Carter-Ruck.

> *It is apparent that, whilst your client's [Wakefield's] letter indeed makes it clear that he "has agreed to help evaluate" some children on behalf of the Legal Aid Board, it does not indicate that in fact such work had been commissioned and was being undertaken before the 1998 Paper was published. In light of this, the* **natural and ordinary meaning**[2] *to be drawn from your client's letter at the time was that following the publication of the 1998 Paper he had agreed to carry out evaluations of children included in the 1998 Paper for the Legal Aid Board.*

Wrong: their "natural and ordinary meaning" is a mundane error that confuses the *present perfect* and *past perfect* tenses. Compounding this error, Olswang's letter continued:

In light of this, and your client's express statement that no conflict of interest existed, our clients had no reason to investigate the position further, until Dr Horton was recently approached by the Sunday Times journalist, Brian Deer. Mr Deer brought to Dr Horton's attention for the first time that your client's relationship with the Legal Aid Board pre-dated the publication of the 1998 Lancet paper by some considerable time.

Apparently, Horton's understanding was that my relationship with Barr had started *after* the 1998 paper was published. In his testimony at the GMC, Horton was to confirm that he believed my relationship with Barr had started "since the publication of the paper" and that because of this, he was prepared to accept that I had no conflict of interest. Moreover, Smith offered Horton clear blue water of "three or four months" between the publication of *The Lancet* paper and the publication of the Rouse letter – easily enough time for Barr and me to have established a working relationship. Let us step back and examine this in a little more forensic detail.

Texas, February 29, 2008. Back at the homestead in Austin, Carmel held the actual Rouse letter — the one that Rouse sent to Horton only **one working day** after the paper's publication. It was labeled LETTLANC. DOC 04/03/98 — referenced by *The Lancet* as having been received on March 4, 1998. *The Lancet* paper was published on Friday, February 28. Rouse's letter was written 1 day later; the weekend came and went, and the letter was faxed to *The Lancet* on Monday, March 4. *The Lancet* faxed this letter, with others, to me on April 2, 1998. Crucially, there are critical differences between the original letter from Rouse and that which was published by *The Lancet* after it had been "edited." The original Rouse letter reads as follows:

Vaccine adverse events: Litigation bias might exist
After reading Wakefield's article I performed a simple internet search and quickly discovered the existence of the society for The Autistically Handicapped. Extracts from this fact sheet are produced below.

*Extracts from a 48 page Vaccines FACT SHEET prepared by Dawbarns for **Society for the Autistically Handicapped** (sic)*

- *Inflammatory bowel disease. We are working with Dr Andrew Wakefield of the Royal Free Hospital. He is investigating this condition. Page 27*

- *Inflammatory bowel disease and autism. If your child has developed persistent stomach problems (including pains constipation or diarrhoea) following the vaccination, ask us for a fact sheet from Dr Wakefield. Page 44*

- *If you believe your child has been damaged...we propose to seek proper compensation in the court. We will also help with applications to the vaccine damage tribunal. Page 47-48*

Rouse provided Horton with a Web address identifying the source of this information.[3] The fact sheet to which Rouse referred Horton carried the date of May 15, 1997[4] — a full 10 months before the paper's publication.

Reading this letter, faxed to me in London by my wife, I was suddenly reminded of Horton's spontaneous denials at the GMC, unprompted by Smith, the prosecuting barrister:

> *To my knowledge in February 1998 and during the peer review process going back into 1997, I was completely unaware of any potential litigation surrounding the MMR vaccine. I was not aware of the involvement of a firm of solicitors Dawbarns. I certainly was not aware of any activity going on with the Society for the Autistically Handicapped prior to the 1998 paper. I was not aware of any other relationship between Dr Wakefield and Dawbarns and Richard Barr.*

This evidence was false. I called Kirsten Limb, a paralegal who, back in the mid-'90s, worked for the plaintiffs' lawyers Dawbarns, the firm that was seeking to determine whether or not there was a case in law against the manufacturers of the MMR vaccine. Kirsten's knowledge of the MMR litigation was and remains encyclopedic, and she was rapidly able to update me on Horton's actual state of knowledge back in 1997. As part of the litigation process, Dawbarns produced fact sheets that were intended primarily for their clients, but requests for copies came from medical practitioners, the pharmaceutical industry, and other interested parties. Over time the fact sheets were updated as further information came to light and the cases progressed.

During the first quarter of 1997, the investigations into *The Lancet 12* were complete and the paper was being written up for submission to the journal. At the same time a Dr. B.D. Edwards wrote to Horton bringing to his attention the fact that text and tables from various *Lancet* papers were being reproduced in Dawbarns's fact sheet, implying breach of copyright.

Limb was telephoned by a Ms. Sarah Quick of *The Lancet.* Limb noted this contact in a memo dated March 19, 1997, marked "Urgent." Quick explained to Limb that Edwards had been in touch and why. A little detective work on Limb's part revealed that Edwards was a member of the Medicines Control Agency (MCA) responsible for vaccine licensing. Apparently, he had chosen not to disclose this fact to Horton by writing to him on his personal stationery.[5] In that telephone conversation, Quick indicated to Limb that Dawbarns should apply to Horton for retrospective permission to reproduce *Lancet* material; she doubted that there would be any problem about the granting of this permission.

Barr duly wrote to Horton explaining the position of Dawbarns. Thorough, as ever, Barr sent his detailed letter by fax and mail on April 3, 1997.[6] In the mailed version, he included his extensive correspondence with a Dr. Wood, also of the MCA (now deceased), and the contentious fact sheet.[7] Barr's letter was explicit: he worked for Dawbarns solicitors, and he was involved in litigation related to potential damage to children following exposure to MMR and MR vaccines. He asked Horton for retrospective permission to quote specific *Lancet* references "contained in the fact sheet," and he identified the four relevant references by providing their footnote numbers in his letter. Footnote number 50 on page 21 of the fact sheet was a reference to a paper that I had coauthored. The text associated with that footnote reads as follows:

> *There is convincing evidence of a link between* [measles] *vaccination and inflammatory bowel disease (including Crohn's disease).*[50] [Footnote 50 is a reference to one of my papers.] *It is a serious lifelong illness that has affected a large number of the children we are helping.* **We are working with Dr Andrew Wakefield of the Royal Free Hospital London. He is investigating this condition.**[8]

For the avoidance of doubt, in March 1997 Barr had taken Horton specifically and deliberately to the text in that fact sheet that described my working relationship with him and his law firm. In the same correspondence, Barr referred specifically to exchanges he had had with me and the fact that I had given him permission to quote papers authored by me and published in *The Lancet.* Intriguingly, in his letter Barr refers to the sinister "pressure from the MCA and the Department of Health on the *Lancet* to have the *Lancet* references withdrawn from the Fact Sheet."

A dialogue started; Horton responded to Barr on April 8, 1997,[9] denying him permission to use material from *The Lancet* in his fact sheet. Barr, clearly frustrated, responded on April 16, 1997, seeking the intercession of *The Lancet's* ombudsman.[10] Horton replied to Barr on April 23, 1997,[11] saying that he would be happy to refer the matter to *The Lancet's* ombudsman. Barr then wrote again to Horton on April 29, 1997,[12] enclosing his correspondence with Dr. Edwards from the MCA and asking to be put in touch with the ombudsman. Horton responded on June 12, 1997,[13] with instructions on how this should be done. Barr acknowledged Horton's letter on June 25, 1997,[14] and subsequently corresponded with *The Lancet's* ombudsman, Professor Sherwood from Cambridge University.[15]

The bottom line is that Sherwood ultimately overruled Horton. He agreed that the tables and other references in the fact sheet could remain, and he indicated that he would be communicating his decision to *The Lancet*. He did so, and Barr heard nothing more from Horton. It would seem reasonable to assume that this correspondence is still held on file by *The Lancet* although, for whatever reason, it was not disclosed to the GMC lawyers when they sought Horton's assistance in my prosecution.

Barr's protracted and contentious exchange with Horton and the subsequent ombudsman's ruling are unusual if not unique in *The Lancet's* history. Beyond any shadow of a doubt, from March 1997 Horton was aware of a number of facts that, in view of the nature and outcome of this exchange, should not have escaped his memory. The material sent directly to Horton at that time included information about Barr, the law firm Dawbarns, the MMR litigation, and my working relationship with Barr and Dawbarns. These, as you will recall from his testimony, were all specifically named and denied by him under oath.

The correspondence concerning breach of copyright started in March 1997 and continued at least into July of that year. Documentary evidence from the GMC indicates that *The Lancet* paper had been submitted for consideration for publication by that time. There appears to have been at least some overlap between the paper's submission and the Barr-Horton-Sherwood exchanges. In my opinion, even if one suspends belief and assumes that Horton had forgotten this exchange, the Rouse letter — sent only days after the paper had been published — and my subsequent confirmation of my role in the litigation would surely have been wake-up calls.

In a nutshell, therefore, it is clear that, as a matter of fact, Horton *was* aware of the law firm Dawbarns, *was* aware of Mr. Barr the lawyer and of his central role in the MMR litigation on behalf of Dawbarns, *was* made aware of my relationship with Barr and my involvement in the litigation — and *all* of this happened one year before the paper's publication. He was reminded of these matters in the Rouse letter and in my response, and was provided with full references to these facts – facts that were never secret – just one working day after the paper was published in February 1998. He was reminded once again by Laurence of *The Independent* newspaper in 2004. Despite all of this, Horton has claimed repeatedly in print, on radio and television, through the law firm Olswang, and under oath upon the witness stand at the GMC, that until 2004 he knew nothing of these matters, claiming instead that he took my response to Rouse to mean that the agreement to work with Barr had started *following* publication of *The Lancet* paper.

This merits a little analysis: Horton appeared to be proposing that **within one working day** of publication (not the 3 to 4 months of clear blue water granted by Smith), Barr and I met, reached an agreement, prepared a fact sheet — for some reason bearing the long-past date of March 13, 1997 — and sent this 48-page document to the Society for the Autistically Handicapped, which duly uploaded it to their website. And all of this was compounded by an apparent amnesia for *his* protracted, contentious, and ultimately luckless exchange with Barr and *The Lancet* ombudsman from March to July of 1997.

A further important contradiction was to arise from Horton's evidence at the GMC when he amplified his false claim of ignorance:

Smith: [Beginning discussion of the Brian Deer meeting on 2/18/04.] *Was that the first you heard of there being an issue?*

Horton: *That is right. That was the first time that I was made aware of the connection, both with the Legal Aid Board and the specific funding of the work that was reported in The Lancet.*

At his meeting with Horton at *The Lancet* offices on the morning of February 18, 2004, Deer alleged that *The Lancet* case series had been funded by the LAB and, therefore, was an actual conflict of interest under the then-applicable disclosure rules of *The Lancet*. I was easily able to refute that allegation during my meeting with Horton later that same day and subsequently confirm at the GMC that the LAB funding was for an as-yet-unpublished viral detection study,[16] while *The Lancet* case series was funded from the Royal Free Hospital and the National Health Service.

Back in 2004, based upon my explanation, Horton immediately retreated from the position of an *actual* conflict to a claim of a possible *perceived* conflict of interest. This led in turn to a heated debate between us, since the then-applicable *Lancet* disclosure guidelines only applied to actual sources of funding, not perceived conflicts. At the conclusion of his evidence at the GMC, Horton confirmed that this exchange reflected a difference in perception and not dishonesty on my part. He confirmed that I was genuinely surprised by his reference to disclosure of a perceived conflict.

The day after this meeting (February 19, 2004), it would appear that Horton reiterated Deer's contention that *The Lancet* paper had been funded by the LAB in a meeting with some of the coauthors at the Royal Free, including pediatric gastroenterologist Dr. Mike Thompson. Thompson gave a statement to the GMC's lawyers, Field Fisher Waterhouse, but, for reasons that are not clear, was not called by them as a witness. His statement reads:

> *In 2004, I met with Richard Horton the Editor of the Lancet along with Dr Murch and Professor Walker-Smith. We were all very shocked to hear about **the funding of the study**[18] and felt very let down by Dr Wakefield. My knowledge about **the funding of the paper**[18] has put the paper into the realms of competing interests. I felt that a retraction of the interpretation of the paper was necessary and a moral obligation.*[19]

So, despite my explanation the previous day, Horton appears to have persisted in Deer's claim that *The Lancet* paper was funded by the LAB. Moreover, Thompson appears to have been motivated to retract the paper's *interpretation* based upon this false premise. However, when Horton came to write his book *MMR: Science and Fiction*[20] the "facts" had changed and he asserted now that, via Deer, he had been aware from the outset of "two quite separate studies":

> *Deer also provided us with evidence suggesting that Wakefield was conducting **two quite separate studies**[21] at the time of publication of his 1998 article. One study included the work that we published in the Lancet. The other investigation was a Legal Aid Board funded pilot project, agreed between the Board and Wakefield in 1996.*

This statement created the appearance that his objection was and always had been based upon a perceived conflict. In this statement he appears to have concealed the fact that it was me, not Deer, who informed him on February 18, 2004, of research — quite separate from *The Lancet* paper — that was funded in part by the LAB. In my opinion, by blurring the crucial distinction between actual and perceived conflicts, Horton made it appear to his readers that he had a reasonable basis for believing that I had failed to make a required disclosure.

In his GMC testimony, Horton was to change his account of this issue once again, admitting that what Deer had, in fact, alleged was that *The Lancet* case series was funded by the LAB:[22]

> **Smith:** *Were allegations – I will deal with them all because you set them out very clearly in The Lancet – did they include allegations in relation to funding issues?*
>
> **Horton:** *Yes, they did.*
>
> **Smith:** *Was that the first you heard of there being an issue?*
>
> **Horton:** *That is right. That was the first time that I was made aware of the connection,* **both with the Legal Aid Board and the specific funding of the work that was reported in The Lancet.**[23]
>
> **Smith:** *How did you handle it, Dr Horton, obviously you listened to what they had to say. What did you do thereafter?*
>
> **Horton:** *Well the presentation by Brian Deer took the form of him standing up before a group of editors and laying out a series of allegations,* **not just relating to the Legal Aid Board funding of the work**[23] *but also including the way the work*[23] *had been handled by the ethics committee at the Royal Free Hospital – two specific allegations, one, that the work had not actually received ethics committee approval and, second, the approval that was given for a piece of work was in some sense a fabrication, that the work that took place and was reported in The Lancet was done under cover of another ethics committee approval process for an entirely different piece of work which was an extraordinarily serious allegation.*

The "work" to which Horton refers is *The Lancet* case series and not the LAB-funded virology study disclosed to him by me (and not by Deer). It is notable that had Horton been accurate about the conflicts of interest issue during the GMC investigation, i.e., that I had, at most, a *perceived* conflict (not a violation of the applicable *Lancet* guidelines), the GMC would not have been able to charge me with an undisclosed *actual* conflict with respect to the LAB funding.

Horton's false testimony was revealed during my evidence. As a result, he was asked to provide an explanation, which he did in a supplemental statement.[24] While he acknowledged that he personally handled the claim in 1997 that Dawbarns infringed *The Lancet's* copyright, he denied having read about my involvement in the litigation. In my opinion, this is most unlikely since he would have had to examine the alleged infringing document personally before deciding whether to grant or deny the requested permission. His denial is limited "to the best of my recollection." His supplemental statement does not obviate in any way the need for a thorough investigation of his actions.

And where is the original Rouse letter? Surely a mundane search of *The Lancet* archives would have revealed it. Horton was first approached by Field Fisher Waterhouse (FFW) in the spring of 2005. They met on March 31 at *The Lancet* offices. Horton reiterated his understanding that the LAB study had been "triggered by the 1998 article being published in February 1998." FFW's attendance note of this meeting continued:

> *Lastly, RH* [Horton] *said he would look for any documents that he might have in relation to this matter.*

This meeting was followed up on June 8, 2005, and opened with Horton inquiring as to whether

> *Dr Wakefield might be able to sue him for defamation should the finalized statement contain any defamatory material.*

This is an odd statement since truth is an absolute defense in defamation. Their meeting concluded as follows:

> [Lawyer]: *I asked RH whether he had found any documents in relation to Dr Wakefield's paper and in particular any private correspondence between The Lancet and Wakefield following the press interest in the article in February 1998. RH said that all[25] of The Lancet documents were archived in the same place and were now stored off site. He had a search done of the archived material and nothing has been found.*

There was no suggestion at any stage that the Rouse letter might have been destroyed. It seems extraordinary, therefore, that what Horton categorically described as a search of archived material containing **all** of *The Lancet* documents, failed to reveal the original Rouse letter – the very letter from which any reference to "litigation bias" and my working with relationship with Dawbarns had been edited.

Postscript

Horton has since issued a full retraction of the 1998 *Lancet* paper on the basis of the GMC's findings. Specifically, he has justified this on the basis of two issues: firstly, the finding that there was no ethical approval for the research described in *The Lancet* paper. This issue is fully addressed in the Afterword, "Ethics, Evidence, and the Death of Medicine."

The second issue is the finding that the description of the children in *The Lancet* paper as "consecutively referred" is false or misleading. This is bizarre, since it is factually entirely correct – these were the first 12 children to be referred to the care of Walker-Smith with a regressive developmental disorder and intestinal symptoms. The paper also adds that these children were self-referred, drawing the reader's attention to the fact that there was this inherent bias in the way cases came to the Royal Free. What has been misconstrued and grossly misrepresented as to the referral process is the fact that parents often made initial contact with me (and I suggested an onward clinical referral to Walker-Smith) and that on a few occasions I spoke to the child's doctor, colleague to colleague, explaining the background to what we thought might be the problem. This process has been portrayed in some way as a corruption of the referral process. But patients and parents frequently make the initial contact with doctors based, for example, on recommendations; doctors often talk to other doctors about complex issues. But the current issue is about protecting MMR vaccine, and that means a whole new set of rules.

It is interesting that the seeds of doubt about the integrity of the referral process were nourished – if not sown – in the minds of the GMC Panel, in my opinion, by none other than Horton himself, ultimately providing a convenient platform from which to issue his full retraction. A medical panel member put it to him:[26]

> *Q: On another issue, what is meant by "consecutive", because in the referrals we talk about consecutive referrals. How do we understand, or what is normally understood, if we see "consecutive referrals" in a paper?*
>
> *A: The ordinary meaning of consecutive referral, to my mind, would literally mean a sequence of children referred one after the other to a*

*specialist, individual or a clinic or unit. That is certainly the way it was presented in this paper. What we found out in 2004, both from what Brian Deer presented to us and also from what Professor Walker Smith discovered and reported to us, was that that consecutive referral, while it was to the letter correct, behind that was actually **a much more complex set of relationships**.*[27]

Since when has the onward referral of sick, non-litigant children whose parents have simply asked for help merited the sinister implication of **"a much more complex set of relationships"**? Horton, in making this allegation, in my opinion, effectively laid the groundwork for a later full retraction of the paper.

In light of factual errors, inconsistencies, and omissions relating to his evidence in the matter of the *GMC vs Wakefield, Walker-Smith, and Murch*, Horton is currently the subject of several complaints to the Professional Conduct Committee of the GMC.[28]

Readers may be interested to know that, in addition to editing *The Lancet* and assisting in the prosecution of me and my colleagues by the GMC, Horton has, since September 2007, been chairing a committee at the Royal College of Physicians in London looking at the relationship between doctors, patients, and the pharmaceutical industry. The deliberations of his group (*Innovating for Health: Patients, Physicians, the Pharmaceutical Industry and the NHS*[29]) were published in February 2009 and have been roundly criticized. The suggestion has even been made that the working party's real agenda was to rehabilitate the image of the drug industry and its relations with clinicians and the NHS. There is a short section on "Medical journals: victims or assailants," which reads as follows:

Editors of medical journals report examples of manipulation, distortion, bias, secrecy, overt promotion, and ghost writing in publishing medical research.

The report goes on to give detailed examples of the "excesses" of industry. What is surprising (or perhaps not) is that the recommendation of the working party does not address the fact that it is unacceptable for drug companies to act in this way but rather the journal editors are asked "to do more to strengthen public and professional confidence." Is this a case of the tail wagging the dog? I cannot say. I wonder, however, whether the ties between *The Lancet*, Elsevier and Glaxo SmithKline – a perceived conflict at the very least – were appropriately disclosed in that report.

Endnotes

[1] Emphasis added.

[2] Emphasis added.

[3] Obtained from http://www.mplc.co.uk/eduweb/sites/autism/index.html Page no longer available.

[4] Dawbarns vaccine fact sheet May 15, 1997.

[5] Correspondence between Edwards and Horton, noted in note of telephone conversation between Sarah Quick (*Lancet*) and Limb (Dawbarns). March 19, 1997.

[6] Barr's fax to Horton of April 3, 1997.

[7] Fact sheet of March 1997.

[8] Emphasis added.

[9] Horton to Barr, Letter April 8, 1997.

[10] Barr to Horton, Letter April 16, 1997.

[11] Horton to Barr, Letter April 23, 1997.

[12] Barr to Horton, Letter April 29, 1997.

[13] Horton to Barr, Letter June 12, 1997.

[14] Barr to Horton, Letter June 25, 1997.

[15] Barr's correspondence with Sherwood, June and July 1997.

[16] *The Lancet* children had completed their investigations by February 1997. Due to the fact that the LAB grant had been placed in a suspense account by Dean Arie Zuckerman, it was not transferred by him to the Special Trustees of the hospital until September 4, 1997, and, therefore, was not available to be spent on the LAB research project until at least September of that year.

[17] *GMC vs Wakefield, Walker-Smith and Murch*, Evidence of Horton Tr. 18, 24.

> **Chairman:** *Coming to the meeting that you had with the three authors who are here, I think you mentioned, which I made a note of, that you told Dr Wakefield that he should have disclosed Legal Aid Board funding?*
>
> **Horton:** *Correct.*
>
> **Chairman:** *What was Dr Wakefield's response?*
>
> **Horton:** *Surprise. He genuinely took the position that he did not see that as a conflict of interest, for the reasons that we have heard, that the Legal Aid Board funding was funding a different study to the one reported in The Lancet, and that he had not considered that something to be worth disclosing to us.*

[18] Emphasis added.

[19] Statement of Dr. M. Thompson to Field Fisher Waterhouse. May 2006.

[20] Horton, R. *MMR Science and Fiction*. London: Granta Books, 2004.

[21] Emphasis added.

[22] *GMC vs Wakefield, Walker-Smith and Murch*, Evidence of Horton Transcript. 17-14D.

[23] Emphasis added.

[24] *GMC vs Wakefield, Walker-Smith, and Murch*. Horton supplemental statement. November 26, 2008.

[25] Emphasis added.

[26] GMC vs Wakefield, Walker-Smith and Murch. Horton Transcript. Tr.18, page 31-32.

[27] Emphasis added.

[28] Complaint of Mr. J. Moody on behalf of various autism organizations, and complaint of Dr. Andrew Wakefield.

[29] Royal College of Physicians. *Innovating for health: patients, physicians, the pharmaceutical industry and the NHS:Report of a working party*. London: RCP, 2009.

CHAPTER NINE

The Devil's in the Detail

The General Medical Council vs. Wakefield, Walker-Smith, and Murch

The research reported by you in *The Lancet* was substantially different from that for which approval was granted by the Ethical Practices Sub-Committee in that it related to:

i) Children with a diagnosis of autism and not disintegrative disorder ...

Your actions were ... inappropriate, not in the best interests of patients, not in accordance with your professional ethical obligations, likely to bring the medical profession into disrepute, and fell seriously below the standard of conduct expected of a registered medical practitioner.

Blake Dobson, Assistant Registrar, General Medical Council

The foregoing is a charge made by the General Medical Council in 2004. The subject matter was "That Paper" – *The Lancet* paper of 1998 that first reported intestinal disease in children with developmental regression. Notwithstanding the fact that in his enthusiasm, Mr. Dobson got the wrong Ethical Sub-Committee approval[1] and the wrong research protocol for the wrong children... there is so much more to this esoteric charge than meets the eye, and the "more" deserves scrutiny. Let's rewind to 1995-7, armed with the enduring adage "if in doubt examine the patient." Among the presenting clinical features of *The Lancet* children were some that were apparently uncharacteristic of autism, at least as it was generally understood at that time. For all 12 children, these included normal or near-normal early development, a clearly delineated onset of behavioral/developmental symptoms, and loss of previously acquired skills. In addition, four children had become incontinent after previously having been potty-trained, while at least six children had developed obvious clumsiness (ataxia), a motor symptom clearly indicative of central nervous system dysfunction (encephalopathy). In contrast with the cold, aloof child described by Kanner, many of these children were affectionate, to the extent that doctors had sometimes been unwilling to make an autism diagnosis.

The combination of these atypical features along with the fact that, for the majority, there was onset following an infectious (vaccine) exposure, led our colleagues in the Department of Child Psychiatry at the Royal Free Hospital to suggest that what we were dealing with was not Kanner's autism, but childhood disintegrative disorder [Panel 1].

Childhood Disintegrative Disorder

In 1908, many years before the publication of Kanner's seminal case series on autism, Theodore Heller, a remedial educator in Vienna, described a new syndrome – *dementia infantilis* (later to become CDD) – in the *Journal for Research and Treatment of Juvenile Feeblemindedness*.[2]

CDD is a pervasive developmental disorder that fulfills behavioral criteria for childhood autism/autistic disorder, but where the pattern of onset is different. CDD requires documented normal or near-normal development[3] up to 24 months of age with subsequent regression and loss of skills in at least two of the following: expressive/receptive language, play, social/adaptive skills, continence, and motor skills [Panel 1].

You might reasonably ask, "But isn't CDD just autism with a later onset and regression?" Later onset following a period of normal development means there are skills to be lost. If the onset occurs after a child is potty-trained, for example, continence may be one of the skills that suffer. And where did 24 months come from? Surely this is entirely arbitrary – an artifact created to satisfy a need to categorize in the absence of a better understanding of the origins of the disease? What do the experts have to say?

- Hill and Rosenbloom noted that "Unlike the vast majority of children with early infantile autism [children with CDD] undoubtedly showed a period of early normal development, including the acquisition of normal language and normal social relationships."[4]

- They observed that the child usually "comes to look very autistic, such that the clinical presentation, but not the history [i.e., regression] is then typical of a child with autism."[3] Rosenbloom cites Professor Sir Michael Rutter as making age of onset a major criterion for diagnosis of CDD[3] in distinguishing it from autism.

- In defiance of Rutter, Malhotra and Gupta[5] noted that "at closer look the age range has varied from 1.2 years (Evans-

Jones and Rosenbloom, 1978) to 9 years (Corbett et al., 1977)."[5] Accordingly, they conclude, "it can be hypothesized that disintegrative disorder [CDD] may be a late-onset variant of autism."

- Russo and colleagues reinforce this view: "Indeed, in many aspects the clinical features [of CDD] are indistinguishable from those of autism, and the differentiating factor is the period of normal early development."[6]

- Malhotra and Gupta noted that "It has been observed that children with CDD have a clearly delineated onset and regression, especially for loss of previously acquired skills, which is absent from autistic disorders."[5]

- The *International Classification of Disease [ICD]-10* itself acknowledges the current "...uncertainty about the extent to which this condition [CDD] differs from autism..."[7]

- The final word goes to Hendry who, in a detailed review of the subject, concluded that "the variables upon which CDD is currently distinguished from Autistic Disorder are not well substantiated."[8] She continued, "CDD should not yet be considered distinct from Autistic Disorder, as not enough information exists to justify it as a separate diagnostic category." Further, she stated that "pervasive developmental disorders could be regarded as a continuum, or spectrum disorder and CDD could be considered a point or range of points along this continuum of behavioural expressions."

In fact, the presenting features of CDD are identical to those of autism with respect to the core symptoms. The key difference lies in the history of normal or near-normal development and regression. The symptoms of CDD fit *The Lancet 12* very well.

So, while opinions differ, any residual distinction appears to hang on the flimsy contrivance of age of onset. For Rutter, as a key prosecution witness at the GMC hearing, however, the matter was black and white. When asked whether "in embarking on a study of children with behavioral disorder, would [he] expect a distinction between CDD and autism to be made," he replied, "Yes." He continued, "and the literature would support drawing a clear distinction at the time [1996]." It is somewhat

---

Panel 1: CDD or Heller's Disease

From around the age of 2 through 10, acquired skills are lost almost completely in at least two of the following six functional areas:

- Language skills
- Social skills & self-care skills
- Control over bowel and bladder

- Receptive language skills
- Play skills
- Motor skills

Lack of normal function or impairment also occurs in at least two of the following three areas:

- Social interaction
- Communication
- Repetitive behavior & interest patterns

---

surprising, therefore, to find that he had earlier written that "The clinical picture [in CDD] after the phase of regression is often somewhat similar to autism and the differentiation may be difficult, **if not impossible**, in cases with an onset before 30 months."[9] It is notable that regression and onset before 30 months applies to virtually all of *The Lancet 12*.

Also notable among the other clinical features of CDD evident in *The Lancet 12* are loss of coordination, secondary incontinence, and, in contrast with "classical" autism, expression of affection.[2,6] Might it simply be that affection, for example, does not make CDD a distinct disease but a different expression of the same disease because, unlike the child with classical autism, the child with CDD has had several years of normal development in which to experience and enjoy affection?

It would seem that Rutter is somewhat isolated in his categorization of childhood developmental disorders by age of onset. Indeed, it is arguably naïve to conceptualize disease in this way, when age of onset may simply better explain differences in presentation. In arguing for splitting autism and CDD, he stated that "although the onset differs from that which is usual in autism, the clinical picture in the two groups of conditions shows many similarities. Nevertheless... for the moment it seems highly desirable to retain [CDD] as a separate category because it is important (a) to recognise that often the syndrome is caused by organic brain disease (b) to appreciate that in some cases the aetiology remains quite unknown; and (c) to accept that the nature and extent of the overlap [with atypical autism] is unknown."[9]

Rutter's reasoning is curious; all three points apply equally to autism – atypical or not – and CDD. Both may be caused by organic brain pathology; in most cases of CDD and autism, the cause is unknown; and, since "the nature and extent of the overlap is unknown," there is little justification for categorizing them separately.

And even now the concept of regression itself appears to be morphing. Whereas, in the past, regression appeared to have been a key distinguishing feature between autism and CDD, Rutter now maintains that regression has always been a common feature of autism.

During his expert evidence at the GMC,[10] Rutter expressed the opinion that for autism "a transient period of regression occurs in 25-30% of cases and is usually temporary." This appears to be at odds with the prior claim that regression was not seen "for the vast majority of children with infantile autism."[4] Rutter may have been referring to temporary loss of language in autism, although this was not clear from his testimony that appeared to focus on *The Lancet 12*.

The data often quoted in support of this position are those of Kurita et al. who reported loss of language in 30% of children with autism.[11] Interestingly, in a second study, Kurita went on to show that the children with regressive autism (the 30% with language loss) were clinically indistinguishable from CDD.[12] In light of their findings, Kurita et al. argued that the validity of CDD being a distinct entity from autistic disorder was unproven and "remains to be studied."

Sadly, for *The Lancet 12*, developmental regression was pervasive – not confined to language alone. Neither was it temporary.

CDD, Autism, and Causation

"If autism is a consequence of vaccination it should have been a consequence of natural infection"

Paul Offit, in interview with Melanie Howard, *Babytalk* magazine

At the heart of the GMC hearing is a defense of the MMR vaccine. Stepping back from the pernicious lies, the political angst, and the cries for blood, it may be valuable to gain some historical vantage point from which to judge scientific concerns about measles virus, vaccines, and developmental disorders. Take for example the presentation of Dr. Daynes to the Royal Society of Medicine in 1956 [Panel 2]. Herein he describes, for all the world, what we see in a clinical setting on a daily basis; apparently there is nothing new.

Panel 2: Measles – bowel – behavior – gluten

Dr. Guy Daynes. Bread and Tears – Naughtiness, depression, and fits due to wheat sensitivity.

Royal Society of Medicine, February 15, 1956

"Typically a child between 1 and 5 years becomes naughty and difficult a few days after the onset of an acute infectious illness... such as measles or gastroenteritis.

"He is irritable, negativistic, and spiteful, sleep is disturbed and he wakes up in the night and often screams; his appetite is poor, he fails to gain weight, his abdomen is often distended and the stools may become bulky, pale and offensive. This condition, if left untreated, usually rights itself after a month or two, but it may last for much longer in which case slight *petit mal* attacks may develop in addition to worsening of the other symptoms.

"I have been placing these children on a gluten-free diet at the earliest opportunity and the symptoms respond dramatically, usually within two or three days. They relapse if a premature return to a normal diet is made.

"Study of over 40 cases has led me to formulate a syndrome – pre-coeliac syndrome."

It is perhaps unsurprising that a further common denominator for some cases of autism and CDD is the causal role of measles virus. This virus, either in its natural or vaccine forms, has been causally linked to childhood developmental disorders, including autism[13-16] and developmental regression.[17]

In utero exposure to measles is associated with autism. Deykin and MacMahon compared exposure patterns of 183 children with autism and

355 sibling controls to the encephalitogenic (causing brain inflammation) viruses, measles, mumps, rubella, and chicken pox. They found that "total autistic symptomatology seems to be associated with prenatal experience with measles and mumps."[13]

In support of a causal role for prenatal measles in autism, Ring et al., used sophisticated statistical modeling of the number of autism births in Israel compared with epidemics of measles, rubella, poliomyelitis, viral meningitis (inflammation of the lining of the brain) and viral encephalitis (inflammation of the brain) and found that peaks in the number of births of children with autism followed peaks of epidemics of measles and viral meningitis.[14]

The authors concluded that "Autistic birth patterns are partially explained by the rates of measles and viral meningitis [incidentally a frequent feature of measles[18]] in the general population. There is a statistically significant environmental association between autism and both viral meningitis and measles that should be further investigated."[14]

CDD has been reported following natural measles infection, and cases have been reported in association with subacute sclerosing panencephalitis, a measles-related encephalitis.[19]

In the case of CDD and measles, Rutter himself wrote that profound regression and behavioral disintegration is often accompanied by a "premonitory period of vague illness, [when] the child becomes restive, irritable, anxious and overactive... Sometimes these conditions come on after measles, encephalitis or other clear-cut organic illnesses."[20]

Among five children who fit the criteria for CDD, Volkmar et al. described a child with onset of behavioral decline following measles encephalitis.[21] Hudolin reported that, prior to regression, a 15-year-old boy with limited speech, stereotyped and repetitive play, and poor self-care skills, etc., suffered from an unknown strain of measles and high fever at approximately 30 months.[22] Malhotra and Gupta confirm that many cases have been associated with some medical condition such as measles.[5]

Vaccines have been associated with CDD; for example, in a report of 12 cases in India seen between 1989 and 1998, Malhotra and Gupta noted onset in four cases with onset following either fever with seizures, acute gastroenteritis, or vaccination. The type of vaccine was not stated.[23]

Dwelling briefly upon the clinical features of ataxia in combination with developmental regression, potentially novel adverse events associated with the combined MMR vaccine, rather than the monovalent component vaccines, have emerged from Plesner's Danish study of ataxia following MMR.[24] Earlier studies had indicated that ataxia with gait disturbance might occur in up to 1 in 1000-4000 recipients of MMR.[25,26] In Denmark this association had not been detected with any other vaccine administered to children of the same age prior to the introduction of MMR in 1987. In a follow-up of the mandatory passive reporting system for vaccine adverse events operated in Denmark, Plesner not only confirmed this association but also indicated that the more severe ataxias following MMR may be associated with residual cognitive deficits in some children,[24] a finding of specific relevance to the MMR-autism debate.

Rutter remains steadfast, however. On behalf of the defendants in US vaccine court and elsewhere, he has taken the position that vaccines are not a cause of autism. Given his pre-eminence, this position is likely to have been highly influential. Meanwhile, the first reported association between vaccines and autism came, not in 1998 with *The Lancet* paper, but in 1993.[27,28] This earlier report took a robust position on the vaccine's likely culpability, certainly compared with the restrained statements in *The Lancet* paper of 1998. In 1993, the authors described 11 children with autism who were excluded from a genetic study based on their having a "medical condition of possible aetiological [causal] importance." The authors stated, "Only eight of the cases can be regarded as having a **probably causal** medical condition, [including] a child with epilepsy and a temporal lobe focus on the EEG who had an **onset following immunization**."[27,28] While the hopes of many desperate parents lie dashed upon the cold marble of the courthouse, it is but an ironic postscript that Professor Sir Michael Rutter, FRS, was the senior author of that paper.

Conclusion

It is proposed that autism and CDD are on the same continuum of clinical disease. Measles virus exposure has been linked to both CDD and autism. The timing of this exposure – i.e., early (*in utero*) or later, in childhood – may determine the clinical presentation, including the presence and extent of regression. Infantile autism without regression may be linked to early exposure, whereas CDD with regression may be linked to later exposure. It is entirely plausible that measles, in combination with two other viruses which have themselves been linked independently to autism – as MMR – may increase the risk for this condition in certain children. Whether or not MMR is guilty as charged remains to be determined.

Endnotes

[1] Ethical Practices Committee (EPC) 172-96 rather than EPC 162-95.

[2] Heller T. Dementia infantilis. *Zeitschrift fur die Erforschung und Behandlung des Jugen lichen Schwansinns.* 1908;2:141-165.

[3] Rutter M. et al. A triaxial classification of mental disorders in childhood. *Journal of Child Psychology and Psychiatry.* 1969;10:41-61.

[4] Hill AE, & Rosenbloom L. Disintegrative psychosis of childhood: teenage follow-up. *Developmental Medicine and Child Neurology.* 1986;28:34-40.

[5] Malhotra S, and Gupta NJ. Childhood Disintegrative Disorder. *Autism and Developmental Disorders* 1999;29:491-498.

[6] Russo M, Perry R, Kolodny E, Gillberg C. Heller syndrome in a pre-school boy. Proposed medical evaluation and hypothesized pathogenesis. *European Child and Adolescent Psychiatry.* 1996;5:172-177.

[7] http://www.who.int/classifications/icd/en/bluebook.pdf

[8] Hendry CN. Childhood Disintegrative Disorder: Should it be considered a distinct diagnosis? *Clinical Psychology Review.* 2000;20:77-90.

[9] Rutter M. *Infantile Autism and Other Pervasive Developmental Disorders in Child and Adolescent Psychiatry: Modern Approaches*; Rutter, M and Hersov, L (1985) Ch. 34, p. 545. Emphasis added.

[10] Testimony of Sir Michael Rutter on behalf of the prosecution. General Medical Council vs. Dr Wakefield, Professor Walker-Smith, and Professor Simon Murch.

[11] Kurita H et al. Infantile autism with speech loss before the age of 30 months. *Journal of the American Academy of Child and Adolescent Psychiatry.* 1985;24:191-196.

[12] Kurita H et al. A comparative study of the development of symptoms among disintegrative psychosis and infantile autism with and without speech loss. *Journal of Autism and Developmental Disorders.* 1992;22:175-188.

[13] Deykin EY and MacMahon B. Viral exposure and autism. *American Journal of Epidemiology.* 1979;109:628-638.

[14] Ring A, Barak Y, Ticher A. Evidence for an infectious aetiology in autism. *Pathophysiology.* 1997; 4:1485-8.

[15] Steiner CE, Guerreiro MM, Marques-De-Faria AP., Genetic and neurological evaluation in a sample of individuals with pervasive developmental disorders. *Arq Neuropsiquiatr.* 2003;61:176-80.

[16] Mouridsen SE, Rich B, Isager T. Epilepsy in disintegrative psychosis and infantile autism: a long-term validation study. *Dev Med Child Neurol.* 1999;41:110-4.

[17] Weibel RE, Caserta V, Benor DE. Acute encephalopathy followed by permanent brain injury or death associated with further attenuated measles vaccines: A review of claims submitted to the National Vaccine Injury Compensation Program, *Paediatrics.* 1998;101:383-387.

[18] Rivinus TM, Jamison DL, and Graham PJ. Childhood organic neurological disease presenting as psychiatric disorder. *Arch Dis Child.* 1975;50:115-119.

[18] Miller HG, Stanton JB, Gibbons JL. Para-infectious encephalomyelitis and related syndromes. *Quarterly Journal of Medicine.* 1956;100:427-445.

[19] Mouridsen SE, Rich B. & Isager T. Validity of childhood disintegrative psychosis: General findings of a long-term follow-up study. *Br J Psychiatry.* 1998;172:263-267.

[20] Rutter M. *Infantile Autism and Other Pervasive Developmental Disorders in Child and Adolescent Psychiatry: Modern Approaches.* Rutter, M and Hersov, L (1985) Ch. 34, p. 556.

[21] Volkmar F. and Cohen DJ. Disintegrative disorder or "late-onset" autism. *Journal of Child Psychology and Psychiatry.* 1989;30:717-724.

[22] Hudolin V. Dementia infantilis Heller; diagnostic problems with a case report. *J Mental Deficiency Research.* 1957;1:79-90.

[23] Malhotra S, Gupta N. Childhood Disintegrative Disorder: Re-examination of the current concept. *European Journal of Child and Adolescent Psychiatry.* 2002;11:108-114.

[24] Plesner AM, Hansen FJ, Taadon K, Nielson LH, Larsen CB, Pedersen E. Gait disturbance interpreted as cerebellar ataxia after MMR vaccination at 15 months of age: a follow-up study. *Acta Paediatrica.* 2000;89:58-63.

[25] Plesner AM. Gait disturbances after measles mumps rubella vaccine. *The Lancet* 1995;345:316.

[26] Taranger J, Wiholm BE. Litet antal biverkninger rapporterade efter vaccination mot massling-passguka-roda hund. *Lakartidningen.* 1987;84:958-950.

[27] Rutter M et al. Autism and known medical conditions: myth and substance. *Journal of Child Psychology and Psychiatry.* 1994;35:311-322.

[28] Rutter et al. (1993) Autism: Syndrome definition and possible genetic mechanisms. In R. Plomin & G.E. McLearn (Eds), *Nature, Nurture and Psychology.* Washington DC: American Psychological Association Press. Emphasis added.

CHAPTER TEN

Bedlam¹ or Bonaparte

I have often wondered where autism might be today had it not fallen into the hands of child psychiatrists. Would things have been very different if, for example, the first child with autism presented before Drs. Gilles de la Tourette,² Joseph Babinski,³ and Pierre Marie⁴ at one of the Tuesday lectures of the great French neurologist Professeur Jean-Martin Charcot?⁵ I think so. Charcot, with his supreme diagnostic skills and clinical intuition, would, I believe, have deferred to his medical training rather than being influenced by the emergent psychoanalysts in his audience.⁶ The debate would have been a brief but interesting one.

While Charcot, known as the "Napoleon of the neuroses," and his colleagues at the Pitié-Salpêtrière Hospital in Paris' 13th arrondissement were limited in their ability to treat the syndromes they described and the diseases they diagnosed, they were, nonetheless, unsurpassed in their ability to take a medical history, observe and elicit physical signs, and ultimately provide us with seminal descriptions of major diseases of the nervous system. Had autism existed in late 19th century Paris, it would doubtless have been described. But it seems these men were unaware of autism as were other equally eminent European and American physicians of the time. Notwithstanding Theodore Heller's report of CDD in 1908,⁷ it was not until 1943 that child psychiatrists first laid claim to autism.⁸ And there it was to remain for many years, an idiosyncrasy, a tragic orphan, a developmental anomaly that left parents without hope or answers. From that time on, it has been a challenging journey – the challenge intensifying as the autism epidemic laid siege to the fondest precepts of this condition. Part of the challenge – not uncommon in the history of medicine – has been the antagonism engendered by different perceptions of a condition, sometimes within the same medical specialty but more commonly between different medical disciplines. This is evidenced by the alternative approaches that different medical specialists have taken to the investigation of autism spectrum disorders.

Part of the controversy at the GMC – an essential element of the prosecution's case against me and my colleagues – was invested in whether or not lumbar puncture (LP), which is often called spinal tap, was an appropriate medical procedure in *The Lancet 12.* The case, played out between their expert, Professor Rutter, and prosecuting counsel was that:

- The children were investigated as part of a research project rather than on the merits of their clinical condition.

- Their clinical condition was not consistent with the symptoms of CDD and, therefore, not compatible with a possible CDD diagnosis.

- Autism – the diagnosis that the majority actually received – does not merit LP.

- Professor Walker-Smith and his team were not capable of making the clinical decision on the merits of undertaking LP.

For good measure, the GMC alleged and the panel ruled that I was guilty of "causing" the children to undergo an LP for the following reasons: 1) I had suggested to concerned parents that, in light of their children's intestinal symptoms, they should seek a referral to Walker-Smith and 2) I had talked with some of the children's doctors either at the parent's or the doctor's request, providing background information. The implications for communication in medical practice are profound.

The first two bullet points above have been dealt with in other parts of this book (see the Afterword, "Ethics, Evidence, and the Death of Medicine," and Chapter 9, "The Devil's in the Detail"). It is the latter two bullet points with which this chapter is concerned, particularly the influence of Rutter on the GMC Panel and, more broadly, the role of medical investigation in children with autism and related disorders in the UK.

LP involves the introduction of a sterile needle between the lower lumbar vertebrae into the space between the lower spinal nerves and their coverings. A sample of the cerebrospinal fluid (CSF) that bathes the brain and spinal cord is withdrawn, placed into a sterile container, and sent to the laboratory for analysis. The procedure is relatively commonplace in the investigation of sick children and is considered by most authorities to carry a minimal risk of complications in experienced hands.[9,10]

LP is undertaken for the purpose of diagnosing inflammation, infection (which may coexist with inflammation), and metabolic abnormalities (derangements of the body's biochemistry). In 1996, metabolic problems amenable to diagnosis by analysis of CSF included mitochondrial disorders (referred to by us in 1996 as "mitochondrial cytopathies"). Congenital or acquired functional defects in the energy factories of the body's cells (mitochondria) are associated with impaired utilization of glucose as an energy source. The body, particularly the brain, relies increasingly on anaerobic metabolism with the accumulation of lactic acid (lactate). This rise in lactate can be detected in spinal fluid, advancing the diagnosis of a possible mitochondrial disorder. In turn, these disorders may be amenable to treatments that boost mitochondrial function and reduce oxidative stress.

Infection as a source of neurological injury in children most commonly takes the form of a relatively rapid-onset event associated with a bacterial or viral infection. On the other hand, with a virus like measles, protracted and persistent infections may occur that have an insidious onset that may be associated with personality change, behavioral problems, and progressive neurological deterioration. Evidence for such an infection may be found by analyzing the CSF. Vaccine-related complications are also relevant in this setting; the meningitis associated with the Urabe AM-9 strain mumps vaccine that led to withdrawal of SmithKline Beecham's *Trivirix* and *Pluserix* MMR vaccines[11] and Aventis Pasteur's *Immravax* MMR vaccine was confirmed by LP and the detection of the mumps vaccine virus in the CSF.[12]

Remaining for the moment with viral infections as a cause of neurological deterioration in children, it is established that various viruses encountered in unusual circumstances are associated with brain damage (encephalopathy), CDD, and − arguably indistinguishable from CDD − autistic regression. These viruses include measles and measles-containing vaccines,[13] mumps and mumps-containing vaccines,[14] rubella,[15] and various *Herpesviridae* including herpes simplex virus type-I,[16] *Cytomegalovirus*,[17] and Epstein-Barr virus (mononucleosis).[18] The unusual circumstances that may allow these historically common viruses to behave in an unusually damaging way may include exposure very early in life, pre-existing immunodeficiency, and immunization. Immunization with three live, modified viruses given together by injection at a much younger age than is typical for natural infection is most certainly an *unusual circumstance*.

Against this background, not all of which was evident to me in 1996, let me characterize the situation that confronted us back then. We encountered a group of children with long-standing intestinal symptoms who, taken at face value, presented with behavioral and developmental regression after a period of normal or near normal early development. The majority had gone downhill shortly after an MMR vaccine. Presented with a highly complex clinical situation, a team of colleagues was brought together under the clinical leadership of Walker-Smith in order to determine what tests were merited for these children with the purpose of shedding diagnostic light on their condition and, thereby, identifying avenues for possible treatment. This – a multidisciplinary clinical collaboration – is exactly what happened, and it worked.

How did the use of LP find its way into the clinical protocol for *The Lancet 12*? First, Dr. Mike Thompson, a pediatric gastroenterologist on Walker-Smith's team and recently arrived from Birmingham Children's Hospital, drew our attention to a clinical protocol developed at that hospital for the investigation of children suffering from neurological deterioration. Mitochondrial disorders were one of the listed diagnoses that needed to be ruled out. The Birmingham protocol advised the use of LP and measurement of lactate in the CSF for this purpose. After reviewing the Birmingham protocol, the children's histories (none had had an LP), and consulting with Dr. Peter Harvey, a clinical neurologist, LP was added to the list of recommended investigations.

Later, under the watchful eye of prosecuting counsel Ms. Sallie Smith at the GMC hearing, Rutter provided a robust dismissal of the merits of LP in the investigation of the majority of *The Lancet 12*. He was substantially less critical under cross-examination by Mr. Adrian Hopkins, QC, senior counsel for Professor Murch, on the issue of investigation for possible mitochondrial disorder[19] – the principal reason for LP in *The Lancet* children.

> **Hopkins:** *What I am putting to you is this: if the Royal Free paediatric gastroenterologists received advice that for children with a history of regression, they should be seeking to exclude mitochondrial disorder and the proper way of doing that was to do a lumbar puncture: that was advice they were reasonably entitled to rely on, is it not?*
>
> **Rutter:** *Yes.*

Second, back at the Royal Free in 1996, a review of the parental narratives led our colleagues in the Department of Child Psychiatry to the provisional opinion that CDD, rather than autism, was the more likely diagnosis in these children. Berelowitz, the lead child psychiatrist, advanced the notion that since his mentor Rutter had reported CDD in association with measles encephalitis (brain inflammation), it was plausible that a measles-containing vaccine might do the same thing. He also pointed out that autism itself may follow congenital rubella (German measles) infection. It was decided, therefore, to look for antibodies[20] to these two viruses in the CSF in order to exclude a long-standing (persistent) brain infection. In light of their history of deterioration following MMR and the knowledge that these viruses can cause chronic brain inflammation with behavioral and developmental regression, you might think it somewhat surprising that this investigation had not been undertaken previously.

Finally, the *research* element of the CSF analyses (for which I was to be responsible) was to look for cytokines — markers of inflammation and immune system activation in the brain. While this test was never done, for reasons that are set out below, it is notable that years later the identification of brain inflammation in autism (neuroinflammation) including abnormal cytokine levels in the CSF was reported by researchers at Johns Hopkins Hospital in Baltimore. Cytokine analysis of CSF has since been used as a clinical procedure in other US centers. This finding has opened up a wholly different view of autism that, combined with the increasing evidence for immunological abnormalities and intestinal inflammation in many affected children, paints an emerging picture of a multisystem inflammatory disorder.

LP in *The Lancet 12*: Clinical or research?

The GMC argued wrongly, but successfully, that LP had been undertaken on *Lancet* children as part of a research agenda, described in ethics committee (EC) application 172-96 (see the Afterword, "Ethics, Evidence, and the Death of Medicine"). Rutter concurred with this on the basis that, in his opinion, there was no clinical justification for LP in these children and that the circumstances of the individual children were not taken into account in prescribing this test.

Discreetly, Rutter had acknowledged from the outset that it would be a "difficult task for the GMC" presumably to find fault with the use of LP in "the clinical treatment" of *The Lancet 12* since, as was revealed in an attendance note from the GMC lawyers,

Some people in America do advocate giving lumbar punctures to children [with autism].[23]

First, let me begin by underscoring the fallacy of the first point. The document labeled by the EC as 172-96 was a clinical *and* research protocol for the investigation of 25 affected children. If LP had been a research procedure, then it would have been undertaken (with parental consent) in all 25 children to be admitted to this study.

For the children reported in *The Lancet*, LPs were stopped on the clinician's instructions after only eight procedures had been performed as it was not yielding any useful clinical information, i.e., information that provided insights into diagnosis and possible treatment.[24] The clinicians made the decision that this clinical test was no longer justified. It is self-evident that if LPs were being performed as part of a research project, then they would have continued in spite of the absence of any clinically positive information because *research* (i.e., measurement of CSF cytokines) rather than clinical care would have been the priority. No measurements of cytokines in CSF were ever undertaken on any of these children; they were *not* part of 172-96. It was decided instead to focus upon the investigation of the intestinal disease that was yielding the most striking and potentially treatable findings. The argument that the children were subjected to an LP for the purpose of research rather than clinical care can be seen to be hopelessly illogical.

Rutter's perception of the evaluation of *The Lancet 12* as research appeared to be motivated largely by an extraordinary attitude toward the investigation of possible vaccine adverse reactions. At the GMC, when shown correspondence between Walker-Smith and a referring physician, he was asked by Smith:[25]

Q: Again, Professor Rutter, is that letter suggestive to you of a research or a clinical investigation?

*A: It sounds much more like a research investigation. It talks about a programme for investigating children. **As for the link with immunisation,**[26] clearly that was a driver for what was being done. That was clear in Mr Wakefield's way of dealing with things, but **that would not be ordinarily seen as a clinical need investigation at that time.**[26] That is the kind of thing that if research had shown a meaningful association, it could become so, but that certainly was not the case at that time.*

Here is an extraordinary admission: in Rutter's opinion, a possible serious adverse vaccine reaction in a child did *not* merit clinical investigation.

This exchange also highlights one of the more substantial planks of the prosecution's case – *inference*: Walker-Smith's reference to a "programme of investigation," sounded more like research to Rutter. In addition, the GMC argued and Rutter concurred that investigation of *The Lancet 12* must have been research since LP was undertaken without a neurologist having seen each child. Rutter ignored the fact that, as well as being specialists in gastroenterology, Walker-Smith and his colleagues are highly experienced pediatricians. LP is a procedure that is prescribed and undertaken by pediatricians on a regular basis. Based upon the clinical evidence available to them, they were entirely capable of making a decision on whether or not LP was appropriate in these children. The *indication* for LP was a *history of developmental regression*. Prior to LP being undertaken, Walker-Smith's team had reassured themselves that there was a history of developmental regression in each of the children on whom this procedure was undertaken.

LP in the investigation of CDD

So what are the merits of LP in a group of children with a suspected diagnosis of CDD? As set out in Chapter 9, "The Devil's in the Detail," there is little, if any, justification for making a distinction between CDD and autism – particularly regressive autism. It is notable, therefore, that LP and analysis of CSF are advocated by many authorities on CDD. Under cross-examination by Murch's senior counsel at the GMC, Adrian Hopkins, QC, Rutter himself advocated the use of LP in *suspected* CDD:[27]

> Q: *If you are faced with a child in whom you suspect true disintegrative disorder as opposed to autism with a regressive element to it, then would you regard it as reasonable to include lumbar puncture in your clinical investigations?*
>
> A: *Yes, I would.*

In a 1996 review of the medical literature and case report by Russo et al.,[28] the authors discuss the key features of CDD and the overlap with autism. In particular, the paper refers to the physical manifestations that accompany developmental decline in affected children. It describes the need for thorough medical and neurological examination of children undergoing acute or subacute deterioration with CDD, including LP and

CSF analysis for measles antibodies to examine for evidence of measles encephalitis. The paper provided useful guidelines for how others might evaluate affected children. The case report goes on to describe CDD with onset at 3.5 years in a boy. The key features in this child's history were:

- normal early development
- progressive loss of vocalization and language
- development of restricted interests
- repetitive behaviors
- secondary urinary and fecal incontinence
- spontaneous inconsolable crying episodes
- loss of self-help skills

Having read Chapter 2, "The Children," the overlap between this child and *The Lancet 12* is evident. Based upon their clinical histories and the advice of our colleagues in child psychiatry, there was every reason to, as in Adrian Hopkins's query, "suspect true disintegrative disorder" in the children who presented to the Royal Free. Other physicians, including Hull – another prosecution witness at the GMC[29] – have also described similar cases and endorsed the approach undertaken by Russo and by Walker-Smith's team at the Royal Free.[30,31] In his textbook, Hull wrote:

> For example, a girl presents at 26 months of age; her development has been quite normal until 20 months of age; her parents then noticed that she had become less responsive and tended to fall more often when walking; over the next 6 months her gait became more unsteady, she played less, her speech regressed and she became irritable. Diagnosis – developmental regression.
>
> **Investigations**
> ...The following list contains only a number of more common and useful investigations ...CSF... elevated protein [and] CSF:serum measles antibody titre ratio...

LP and autism

The role of LP in autism is more contentious than for CDD, and expert opinion is sharply divided. In fact, debate over the merits of this procedure reflects, in some ways, the larger debate over the priority of genetics or environment in this disorder. Rutter, as an advocate for the genetic basis of autism, sees relatively little merit in routinely investigating its possible organic basis in detail, even though he acknowledges the organic basis of the disorder.[32] In fact, in his report to the GMC lawyers he wrote:

> *I know of no child psychiatrist or child neurologist in the UK who would regard lumbar puncture as a justifiable routine investigation of children with an autism spectrum disorder. Both would be aware that **periods of regression are very common in autism**[34] and are not an indication for detailed invasive investigation.*

Alternatively, Christopher Gillberg, a professor of child and adolescent psychiatry and autism expert from Sweden, advocates LP in the routine clinical investigation of children with autism, and in his hands, when specific hypothesis-testing studies have been performed on CSF, these have consistently identified differences between children with autism and non-autism controls that support the likelihood of an underlying organic pathology.[35]

Rutter portrayed Gillberg's experience somewhat differently in his GMC testimony. When asked by Smith whether Gillberg's published findings advocated LP in autism, Rutter was dismissive:[36]

> *As far as I know he still advocates doing so, but what is quite striking in the published reports is the absence of any evidence that it is actually useful.*

Under cross-examination by Hopkins, Rutter put it more strongly:[37]

> *The evidence from Gillberg or any of the other people who use this approach is absolutely consistent in its negativity … So Gillberg's own findings actually run counter to the advice that he gives.*

In fact, Rutter's antipathy toward Gillberg was a recurring theme in his evidence, which at one time described him as having

> *…an unenviably high reputation for findings that could not be replicated.*

Rutter's recurring disdain for his colleague earned him rebuke under cross-examination. When Hopkins brought Rutter's attention back to the fact that Gillberg's analysis of CSF had actually led to a series of positive, published findings, Rutter defaulted to a dismissal of Gillberg's science in general.

The GMC Panel was led to believe that the use of LP was a peculiarly Swedish – indeed, peculiarly a Gillberg – phenomenon. During Hopkins's cross-examination, he pointed out to Rutter that Gillberg had coauthored an authoritative textbook with Dr. Mary Coleman, a pediatric neurologist from the US, in which they had written:[38]

...lumbar puncture is there to exclude progressive encephalitis and encephalopathy...

*...the evidence concerning the association, even of so called classical autism cases, with a wide variety of specific medical conditions, ... is now such that it must be considered **clinically unacceptable not to perform a work-up of this kind.**[39]*

The challenge to Rutter from both sides of the Atlantic was clear – his diagnostic approach to autism was, in Gillberg and Coleman's opinion, "unacceptable."

This professional hostility appears to have been part of a long-standing debate over whether or not a more thorough clinical investigation of children with autism increases the yield of medical disorders and, therefore, potential opportunities for treatment.

Does more thorough investigation of children with autism increase the yield of medical diagnosis?

In 1996, Gillberg and Coleman[40] provided a comprehensive review of the association between autism and medical disorders based upon seven population-based studies. They wrote:

The rate of associated specific medical disorders and/or organic conditions in autism has varied from 11 or 12% in population-based studies that did not include comprehensive neurological and medical investigation (Gillberg 1984[41]: Rivto et al. 1990[42]) to 37% in studies that did include such investigation (Steffenburg 1991[43]). In the latter study, only 17% would have been shown to have an associated medical disorder if the neuropsychiatric assessment had not been comprehensive. Thus it seems that the more comprehensive the medical examination, the greater the yield of associated medical disorders.

Intuitively, it would seem to be of fundamental importance to identify associated medical disorders, in particular, where such disorders lead to the possibility of effective treatments; an example of this would be herpes virus encephalitis. Gillberg and Coleman were critical of Rutter and his colleagues based upon what they consider to be a fundamental error in

Rutter's analytical approach to the available studies:

Some authors (e.g. Bailey 1993[44]. Rutter et al 1994[45]) appear to believe that the rate of associated medical disorders can be compared across studies regardless of the representativeness of the sample or the comprehensiveness of the examination. Since almost all autism studies (often on clinic or otherwise referred patient groups rather than community-based samples) have included only very limited medical investigation (physical examination plus chromosome, blood and urine screens at most), the conclusion has been that associated medical disorders, although occurring in a proportion of autism cases, are relatively rare (around 10 to 12% according to Rutter et al. 1994).

In the published literature, however, the only population-based autism sample to receive a comprehensive medical, biochemical and neurological examination was the one reported by Steffenburg (1991). The Wing and Gould (1979) study was probably the next most comprehensive study in this respect, and the overall prevalence of possibly autism-related medical disorders was almost identical. Therefore, until other population-based samples have been subjected to comprehensive medical examination (which is not to be equated with a range, however wide, of blood and urine tests only), it remains open to speculation just how large the proportion of cases with associated medical disorders is.

They continued:

...regardless of whether the rate of associated medical disorders in autism is 11%, 24%, or 37%, there is clearly a need for a comprehensive medical examination. Several of the medical disorders that are now known to be sometimes associated with autism can only be diagnosed by extensive examination, which should include... cerebrospinal fluid examination (for encephalitis and progressive encephalopathies).

Here we have well-recognized authorities on autism making a strong case for the routine use of LP in the diagnosis of medical disorders associated with autism. From the Institute of Psychiatry, King's College London, in 2001, another of Rutter's protégés, Dr. Patrick Bolton, acknowledged both sides of the medical investigations debate when he wrote:

The choice of appropriate tests to identify these conditions has to be guided by the history and results of physical examination, as well as the expected yield and invasiveness of the procedure. This has been the subject of some debate in the investigation of children with autistic spectrum disorders, with some clinicians advocating that an extensive medical work up (e.g. brain scans and lumbar punctures) always be conducted (Gillberg and Coleman, 1996). By contrast, the majority favour a much more limited set of investigations (Rutter 1994; Barton and Volkmar 1998).[47]

However, Bolton makes no reference to the fact that the diagnostic yield of associated medical conditions is substantially increased by the approach advocated by Gillberg and Coleman. Bolton continued:

The likelihood of identifying a medical condition is related to the severity of the developmental disorder and is greatest in people with severe and profound degrees of handicap

If this was intended to aid others in identifying subgroups of children (i.e., those with profound degrees of handicap) that should undergo more extensive medical investigation, then it fails to provide adequate guidance. Bolton also fails to mention that the likelihood of identifying a medical condition is directly related to the diligence with which it is sought. In contrast with the rather nihilistic view of Rutter and colleagues, Dr. Cheryl Hendry from the University of Georgia advocates that

There is also a significant need to clarify the nature of possible organic causes of CDD, Autistic Disorder, and other pervasive developmental disorders, as well as the mechanisms of neurological insult.[48]

The most effective way to do this is to adopt a more aggressive, systematic approach to delineating the organic basis of the symptoms in each and every child. Rutter's 1994 paper[50] is instructive when he states:

Gillberg has urged that the supposed strong association with known medical conditions means that extensive investigations including lumbar puncture and CAT scan should be undertaken as routine. Federico et al (1990) have put forward similar arguments... However, most reviewers have not considered lumbar puncture or brain imaging as part of the range of essential investigations to be undertaken in the absence of specific indications (Rutter 1985; Bailey 1994).

Rutter does not provide an explanation of what these "specific indications" might be until somewhat later in the paper when he states:

It seems very dubious whether it is necessary to perform a lumbar puncture in the absence of any clinical indications of deterioration.

It seems, therefore, that "deterioration" in the condition of a child is an indication for LP. All 12 of the children reported in *The Lancet* exhibited deterioration. Furthermore, under the rubric of Rutter's "specific indications," it has been considered routine, i.e., *standard of care*, to examine CSF in children when their autistic regression has been associated with a specific infectious exposure.[51] It seems logical to assume that the chance of identifying a causative infection is likely to be much greater when developmental regression follows a documented infectious (or vaccine) exposure. And yet, when a child's deterioration follows a *vaccine* – one containing viruses that are well known to be capable of infecting the brain, causing inflammation, and have been associated with autism in the medical literature – LP is frowned upon to the extent that it becomes a charge of medical misconduct.

Moving on from Rutter and child psychiatry, what is the opinion of experts in child neurology who, in contrast with many psychiatrists, are more invested in the organic basis of nervous system disease rather than its possible psychological origins? The late Dr. John Menkes, professor emeritus of neurology and pediatrics at UCLA and editor of the definitive textbook *Child Neurology*, was a world authority on autism and related disorders. Exclusion of mitochondrial cytopathy by measurement of CSF lactate is described specifically by Dr. Menkes as an indication for the procedure in such children.[52] In an e-mail to me on February 11, 2006, shortly before his death, he added:

It is my opinion, and we so expressed it in the latest edition of my textbook, a CSF analysis can "assist" in the differential diagnosis of regressive autism. It is also my opinion that the risks of a lumbar puncture in a child with autism are so miniscule that I see no contraindication to the procedure.

Dr. Marcel Kinsbourne is a pediatric neurologist and an expert in childhood developmental disorders. He trained in medicine at Oxford University and Guy's Hospital in London and is currently an emeritus professor of pediatric neurology at Tufts University in Boston. His expert opinion is as follows:

When a child who has hitherto developed normally, begins to lose mental skills progressively in the second year of life, this represents a progressive encephalopathy that requires diagnosis. The fact that the final outcome of the regression takes the form of the behavioral syndrome of autism is of little diagnostic help as it is well known and generally agreed that there are at least dozens of different causes of syndromes of the autistic spectrum. Specifically such a child could have a degenerative metabolic or a subacute inflammatory condition of the nervous system, for instance as caused by a "slow virus". If that were the case, it would be important to establish this for purposes both of prognosis and potential treatment.

The most direct way of determining the medical condition of the brain, short of brain biopsy, which would be inadmissible in most such cases, is to study the composition of the cerebrospinal fluid. Abnormal cytology and markers of infection such as immune globulins, the infectious agent itself or fragments of its genome can nowadays be detected with high sensitivity. The spinal fluid is acquired through lumbar puncture (spinal tap). In my chapter in Textbook of Child Neurology *(Menkes, Sarnat & Maria, eds, 2006), I write as follows in the section entitled "Autism: Diagnostic Evaluation": "A spinal tap can assist in the differential diagnosis of new onset seizures or autistic regression" (page 1118).*

To study a child who has regressed from normal development into an autistic syndrome by lumbar puncture is not in the least abusive; it is thoroughly warranted on clinical grounds.[54]

The UK's experience with mad cow disease (bovine spongiform encephalopathy or BSE) has been a timely instruction in the correct approach to neuropsychiatric syndromes of unknown cause. Martin Rossor, professor of clinical neurology at the National Hospital for Neurological Diseases and St. Mary's Hospital, London, gave the following evidence to the UK's *Southwood* BSE enquiry on October 26, 1998:[55]

The differential diagnosis of patients presenting with cognitive disturbance, particularly in the young, is very wide. Such patients require careful assessment and extensive investigation.

He continued:

Neuro-imaging should be undertaken in the majority of patients presenting with cognitive impairment and it is mandatory in all unusual cases and all young people... All unusual and young onset patients with dementia should also have the cerebrospinal fluid (CSF) examined by lumbar puncture. This will identify inflammatory changes suggesting an infection or inflammatory disorder such as multiple sclerosis.

So, you appreciate that there is, at the very least, a divergence of expert opinion on the merits of LP in the investigation of autism. There is less when the autism is regressive and no debate over the need for LP in the investigation of CDD. You might think that the appropriate forum for the resolution of any outstanding differences would be the pages of medical journals rather than from the witness stand of the GMC.

Where are we now?

LP was abandoned in early 1997 as a routine clinical procedure in the affected children presenting to the Royal Free. In the small number of children who had this investigation, it did not reveal any evidence of a mitochondrial disorder, nor were antibodies against measles and rubella present in the CSF. Under these clinical circumstances, Walker-Smith and his team decided to pull this test in order to reduce the number of procedures the children underwent.

Mitochondrial disorders have since become a hot topic in autism with a high proportion of children showing evidence of mitochondrial dysfunction[56] – something that they may have been either born with or acquired from an environmental stressor early in life, such as organic mercury. Nonetheless, there have been advances in diagnostic techniques, and LP is not necessarily required to detect mitochondrial disorders.

In hindsight with respect to looking for a possible viral cause, it may be that stopping LPs at the Royal Free was premature. When we undertook a more detailed analysis of CSF on three similarly affected US children in collaboration with Dr. James Jeffrey Bradstreet of Florida and Professor John O'Leary of Dublin, the same unique parts of measles virus genetic material were found in the CSF of all three children.[57] In addition, elevated levels of measles antibody were found in two of the three children. No evidence of measles virus was found in the CSF of three non-autism control children. The laboratory techniques for measles gene detection in O'Leary's lab have since been criticized[58] and vindicated.[59] A larger study using the same technology was later presented at a scientific meeting on autism;[60] submission of the full publication has awaited resolution (successful) of the technical issues associated with measles virus detection.

The Methods section of the draft paper explicitly states the clinical indication for undertaking the procedure in children with autistic disorder:

Since AE [autistic encephalopathy] children had suffered neurological deterioration associated with developmental regression following a viral exposure, CSF analyses were therefore clinically indicated in the presence of an incompletely diagnosed regressive encephalopathy.

In this study, measles virus genetic material was present in CSF from 19 of 28 (68%) cases and in one of 37 (3%) non-autism controls. Further tests confirmed that where there was sufficient amount of sample available, the genetic material was consistent with having come from the vaccine virus.

The draft paper concludes by saying,

*The data indicate that virological analysis of CSF is indicated in children undergoing autistic regression following **exposure**[61] to live vaccine viruses.*

The paper's conclusions stop well short of any claim that the MMR vaccine causes autism. The most one can say from the findings of measles viral genetic material in CSF is that there is a strong statistical association between the presence of this virus and the autism group. The finding of measles antibody in CSF in the smaller study is in some ways more interesting since it suggests local production of an immune response to measles virus in the brain of some affected children. Further study is clearly required to see if this finding can be replicated elsewhere.

What is the current status of genetics? Substantial – almost exclusive – investment in a genetic model of autism has lead to disappointment, to say the least. Genetic studies have comprehensively failed to substantiate any belief that for the great majority of cases autism represents a primary genetic disorder. Rather, the prevailing consensus is that the majority of current autism cases occur in response to a variety of environmental causes or triggers to which there may be a genetic predisposition. But this is where the bias of so many experts in the field resides. Lauding the child psychiatrist who first described autism, Rutter wrote this of Kanner:

In an era that has sometimes been thought of representing "epidemic environmentalism", he was astute in suggesting that autism represented some kind of inbuilt deficit.

One cannot help but feel that this bias in so influential a body of experts has restricted their viewpoint to the extent that progress has been impeded.

The necessary transition for many diseases from the genetic model to a dominant environmental model is not a new one. Until the 1980s, immunodeficiency syndromes were relatively rare, consisting of a mixed bag of genetic anomalies that compromised various aspects of immunity, leading to opportunistic infections and cancer. Then they were not; an epidemic of acquired immunodeficiency dropped people in their thousands as AIDS swept the globe. As another instance, I remember only too well lectures in the 1980s on the relationship between the genetics of blood groups and the associated risk of duodenal ulcers, stomach ulcers, and stomach cancer. An Australian doctor refocused the attention of the medical community on a helical bacterium in the stomach of ulcer sufferers, treated them with antibiotics, and cured their ulcers. That was the end of any discussion of blood group genetics. This is not to say that it was wrong; it just became redundant, irrelevant in the face of a far more compelling set of facts. Autism is currently undergoing the same transition.

And before overfocusing on the categorical delineation of one set of children from another based upon their presenting features, it should be borne in mind that the manifestations of environmentally-driven diseases will be determined to a large extent by the pattern of exposure to the causal environmental factor(s). Variables that matter include how old you are when you get "hit," what dose you get hit with, if you are coincidentally ill with another disease when you get hit, what your genetic predisposition is, and by what route of exposure you are hit. In the context of the vaccine debate, the nature of sequential or concurrent exposures to the likes of mercury and aluminum that modify immune responses, and live viral vaccines whose behavior is dependent on those immune responses will, I believe, be a major determinant of what an adverse reaction looks like.

A causal exposure at 6 months of age may cause an autistic syndrome that leaves a child asocial, lacking speech and language, always incontinent, and classically autistic. In contrast, the same exposure at 3 years of age may cause the same child to lose speech and language, lose previously acquired continence, but remain affectionate to those he knows because he has learned the rewards of shared affection; now his disorder will receive a label of atypical autism or CDD. In this example, the different manifestations of the same disease process should not be artificially distinguished as has been advocated for autism and CDD according to Rutter's major criterion of age-of-onset. To do so implies that they have different causes; the clues are missed, and the disease and its cause(s) end up chasing — but never catching — the artificial labels.

Child psychiatry has applied itself most comprehensively to the description and subcategorization of autistic disorders, drawing and redrawing the lines that apparently distinguish some affected children from others. The fifth iteration of the *Diagnostic and Statistical Manual of Mental Disorders* (DSM-V) from the American Psychiatric Association is in preparation,[62] redrawing these lines once more. The need to do this is driven, in part, by the changing presentation of autistic disorders themselves, e.g., the increasing frequency of autistic regression. One should not underestimate the importance of this descriptive process, for which Rutter must take much of the credit. It's simply that, from the perspective of *this* outsider, such a self-perpetuating process means that the actual disease (and by extension, its cause[s]) ends up chasing the definitions rather than the other way around.

As a discipline, child psychiatry has been far less helpful in guiding doctors on how to investigate affected children. Gillberg was candid about these shortcomings when he wrote:

> *There is a very conspicuous lack of literature in the field of autism work-up. Guidelines for clinicians planning to work up their patients with autism are virtually nonexistent.*[63]

Finally, there is a different way of looking at disease; one that discards categorization with the end point determination of whether a child fulfills the diagnostic criteria for a full-blown autism diagnosis or falls just short with a label of pervasive developmental disorder – not otherwise specified (PDD-NOS). This alternative approach does not *just* start with the parental narrative – it is truly invested in it, using it as the navigation system without which the disease is condemned to forever wander in the wilderness of psychiatric name-calling. There is no room for bias, prejudice, or recrimination in this medical model. The overspecialized doctor must be prepared to embrace the *New*, revisit the medical school lessons in immunology and biochemistry, embrace rather than fear change – particularly for a condition where such ignorance prevails, and not run when parents mention vaccines as a possible trigger. There is no more complex a disease than that seen in the autistic children who attended the Royal Free – children that the prosecuting counsel at the GMC claimed were not actually sick at all . . . children that some at the Royal Free actively turned away – God help them. But the starting point is easy – humbling in the face of so much that is unknown; it is the parents' story. That does not mean that disease will give up its secrets easily, but it's a start.

I return to that first child for whom Rutter described immunization as the "probable" cause of his autism as I described for you in Chapter 9, "The Devil's in the Detail."[64] Clearly, Rutter and his coauthors acknowledged the validity of the parental narrative and documented it in strong terms. With this history of onset following vaccine exposure, what did Rutter consider to be the mechanism of damage that led this child into autism? And how was this child investigated? Having described this case in 1994, in the early years of the UK's autism epidemic and well into it in the US, this would have provided a very important insight. With Rutter's gravitas behind it, who knows what impact this might have had in shaping perception and the research agenda. But unfortunately, as is evident from Rutter's testimony under cross-examination in US vaccine court[65] the child's history seems to have left little impression on him.

> *Q: Now, you're actually discussing in this paragraph a review paper that you had published, actually a study you had published back in 1993 on Systematic Investigation of 100 Individuals With Autism. And you say here that only eight of these cases can be regarded as having probably a causal medical condition, one being a child with epilepsy and temporal lobe focus on the EEG who had an onset following immunization. Do you see that?*
>
> *A: (Nonverbal response.)*
>
> *Q: I assume that that was a case of regressive autism, wasn't it?*
>
> *A: I have no memory as to whether it was or it wasn't. I'm sorry. I can't help you on that.*

And what about the comorbid gastrointestinal problems in children with autism; are they new or were they there all along, languishing while the collective dissonance of the *cognoscenti* defaulted to an attitude of "that's just autism for you"? Kanner described gastrointestinal symptoms in a high proportion of his first patients;[66] Dohan and Goodwin described such symptoms in 1968 and 1971, respectively;[67] Walker-Smith reported them in 1972;[68] Gillberg and Coleman sought to highlight "celiac autism" as a subtype in their textbook in 1985;[69] there is nothing new.

And Rutter — where does he stand in all of this? Under cross-examination from Stephen Miller, QC, leading counsel for Professor Walker-Smith, Rutter was asked about gastrointestinal symptoms in autism.

A: I think it is something certainly well worth looking at. The general proposition, just to return to that for a moment, is that individuals with autism frequently have GI symptoms. That is uncontroversial and clear. It would be of potential value to understand what on earth that means. I agree with that. Therefore the investigation of those in more detail I would certainly support. [70]

Despite this, it was evident from further questioning that Rutter had had no collaborative interaction with a pediatric gastroenterologist in either a clinical or research setting. Since Rutter acknowledged that intestinal symptoms are so "common and uncontroversial"[71] in patients with autism, this begs the simple question, "why not?"

I am left wondering how those doctors at the Pitié-Salpêtrière would have viewed the gastrointestinal symptoms and their potential link to disordered neurology in autism. As it is, in some corner of the Cimitière de Montmartre, Paris, Charcot is likely to have turned in his grave several times in the light of what has befallen these children. Ultimately, it took a group of gastroenterologists to recognize the significance of these symptoms, not through some preternatural wisdom, but through the diligent application of their training. A new syndrome was described and the findings replicated around the world.[72] Erasure from the Medical Register is a small price to pay for the privilege of working with affected families.

Endnotes

[1] Bethlehem Psychiatric Hospital (Bedlam) in the London borough of Bromley, where Professor Sir Michael Rutter, FRS, and his colleagues worked in the Department of Child Psychiatry.

[2] Georges Albert Édouard Brutus Gilles de la Tourette (1857-1904) was a French neurologist who described what became known as *Tourette syndrome* in nine patients in 1884 as *"maladie des tics."* Charcot gave the syndrome the eponymous title *"Gilles de la Tourette's illness."*

[3] Joseph Jules François Félix Babinski (1857-1932) was a Polish neurologist. In 1896, he described what became known as Babinski's sign, a pathological plantar reflex (upward movement of the toes elicited by stroking the sole of the foot (*"phenomène des orteils"*) indicative of central nervous system (*corticospinal tract*) damage.

[4] Pierre Marie (1853-1940) was a French neurologist who, among other things, described a disorder of the pituitary gland known as acromegaly, an overproduction of growth hormone leading to "giantism."

[5] Jean-Martin Charcot (1825-1893), "the Napoleon of the neuroses," was a French neurologist and professor of anatomical pathology. He is one of the pioneers of neurology, and his name is associated with at least 15 medical eponyms, including joint manifestations of neurosyphilis, Charcot-Marie-Tooth disease, and amyotrophic lateral sclerosis (Lou Gehrig's disease).

[6] Sigmund Freud went to Paris in 1885 to study with Charcot.

[7] Theodore Heller, a special educator in Vienna, proposed the term *dementia infantilis* in 1908 to account for the condition of developmental regression described in "The Devil's in the Detail."

[8] Kanner L. Autistic disturbances of affective contact. *Nerv. Child.* 1943;2:217-50.

[9] The late Professor John Menkes, Department of Neurology, UCLA, to AJW via e-mail of February 11, 2006: "It is also my opinion that the risks of a lumbar puncture in a child with autism are so miniscule that I see no contraindication to the procedure."

[10] GMC vs. Wakefield, Walker-Smith and Murch. Rutter testimony: Tr. 38.
   Q. [Hopkins] *Lumbar puncture for CSF analysis is a safe and relatively non-traumatic procedure.*
   I think you agree with that proposition?
   A. [Rutter] *Yes.*

[11] The same vaccine withdrawn as *Trivirix* in Canada and launched in the UK as *Pluserix.*

[12] See Chapter 4, "The Whistleblower," and Martin Walker's article titled "The Urabe Farrago." Retrieved from: http://www.wesupportandywakefield.com/documents/The%20Urabe%20Farrago.pdf

[13] Weibel RE, Caserta V, Benor DE. Acute encephalopathy followed by permanent brain injury or death associated with further attenuated measles vaccines: a review

of claims submitted to the national vaccine injury compensation program, *Pediatrics.* 1998;101:383-387.
Deykin EY, MacMahon B. Viral exposure and autism. *American Journal of Epidemiology.* 1979;109:628-638.
Ring A, Barak Y, Ticher A. Evidence for an infectious aetiology in autism. *Pathophysiology.* 1997;4:1485-8.

[14] Johnstone JA, Ross CAC, Dunn M. Meningitis and Encephalitis Associated with Mumps Infection: A 10-Year Survey. *Arch Dis Child* 1972;47:647-651.

[15] Chess S. Autism in children with congenital rubella. *J Autism Dev Disord.* 1971;1:33-47.

[16] DeLong RG, Bean C, Brown F. Acquired reversible autistic syndrome in acute encephalopathic illness in children. *Child Neurology.* 1981;38:191-194.
Gillberg C. Brief report: onset at age 14 of a typical autistic syndrome. A case report of a girl with herpes simplex encephalitis. *J Autism Dev Disord.* 1986;16:369-375.

[17] Stubbs EG, Ash E, Williams CPS. Autism and congenital cytomegalovirus. *J Autism Dev Disord.* 1984;14:183-189.

[18] Shenoy S, Arnold S, Chatila T. Response to steroid therapy in autism secondary to autoimmune lympho-proliferative syndrome. *J Pediatrics.* 2000;136:682-687.

[19] GMC vs Wakefield, Walker-Smith and Murch. Tr.38 page 20.

[20] Immune system proteins that specifically target and protect the individual from invading infections. Antibodies are found in the blood and at the mucosal surfaces of the body such as the lung and intestine

[21] Vargas DL, Nascimbene C, Krishnan C, Zimmerman AW, Pardo CA. Neuroglial activation and neuroinflammation in the brain of patients with autism. *Ann Neurol.* 2005;57:67-81.

[22] Department of Neurology, the Chicago Medical School of Rosalind Franklin University; the Sutter Neuroscience Institute in Sacramento; and the Department of Educational Psychology at Illinois State University. See: M. Chez, T. Dowling, P. Patel, P. Khanna, M. Kominsky. Elevation of Tumor Necrosis Factor-Alpha in Cerebrospinal Fluid of Autistic Children. *Pediatric Neurology,* 2007;36:361-365. "The current procedure [LP] was elective and was done to exclude a degenerative process. The patients had routine clinical cerebrospinal fluid studies performed including cell count for red and white blood cells, total protein and glucose levels."

[23] GMC vs Wakefield, Walker-Smith, and Murch. Attendance note from unused material Rutter to Field Fisher Waterhouse. September 7, 2006.

[24] AJW letter to Pegg. February 3, 1997.

[25] GMC vs Wakefield, Walker-Smith and Murch. Rutter Testimony Tr 35. p.56.

[26] Emphasis added.

[27] GMC vs Wakefield, Walker-Smith and Murch. Rutter Testimony Tr. 38. Page 25.

[28] Russo M, Perry R, Kolodny E, Gillberg C. Heller syndrome in a pre-school boy. Proposed medical evaluation and hypothesized pathogenesis. *European Child and Adolescent Psychiatry.* 1996;5:172-177.

[29] Hull D and Milner AD. *Hospital Paediatrics.* London. Churchill Livingston, 1984.

[30] Mouridsen SE et al. A comparative study of genetic and neurobiological findings in disintegrative psychosis and infantile autism. *Psychiatry and Clinical Neurosciences.* 2000;54:441-445.

[31] Malhotra S and Gupta N. *J Autism Dev Disord.* 1999;29:491-498.

[32] Rutter et al. Autism and known medical conditions: myth and substance. *J. Child Psychol. Psychiat.* 1994;35:311-322.

[33] Rutter report to Field Fisher Waterhouse. May 7, 2007.

[34] Emphasis added.

[35] Gillberg C, Terenius L, Hagberg B, Witt-Engerstrom I, Eriksson I. CSF beta-endorphins in childhood neuropsychiatric disorders. *Brain Dev.* 1990;12:88-92.
Ahlsen G, Rosengren L, Belfrage M, Palm A, Haglid K, Hamberger A, Gillberg C. Glial fibrillary acidic protein in the cerebrospinal fluid of children with autism and other neuropsychiatric disorders. *Biol Psychiatry.* 1993;15:734-43.
Gillberg C, Svennerholm L. CSF monoamines in autistic syndromes and other pervasive developmental disorders of early childhood. Br J Psychiatry. 1987;151:89-94.
Gillberg C. Not less likely than before that mean CSF HVA may be high in autism. *Biol Psychiatry.* 1993; 15;34:746-7.
Nordin V, Lekman A, Johansson M, Fredman P, Gillberg C. Gangliosides in cerebrospinal fluid in children with autism spectrum disorders. *Dev Med Child Neurol.* 1998;40:587-94.
Vargas DL, Nascimbene C, Krishnan C, Zimmerman AW, Pardo CA. Neuroglial activation and neuroinflammation in the brain of patients with autism. *Ann Neurol.* 2005;57:67-81.

[36] GMC vs Wakefield, Walker-Smith and Murch. Rutter Testimony. Tr. 35. p23

[37] GMC vs Wakefield, Walker-Smith and Murch. Rutter Testimony. Tr. 38. p22

[38] GMC vs Wakefield, Walker-Smith and Murch. Rutter Testimony. Tr. Day 35. P22

[39] Emphasis added

[40] Gillberg C and Coleman M. Autism and medical disorders: a review of the literature. *Dev Med and Child Neurol.* 1996;38:191-202.

[41] Gillberg et al. Infantile autism and other childhood psychoses in a Swedish urban area. *J Child Psych and Psychiat.* 1984;25:35-43.

[42] Ritvo et al. The UCLA–University of Utah epidemiologic survey of autism: the etiologic role of rare diseases. *Am. J Psychiat.* 1990;147:1614-21.

[43] Steffenburg S. Neuropsychiatric assessment of children with autism: a population based study. *Dev Med Child Neurol.* 1991;33:495-551.

[44] Bailey A, et al. Prevalence of Fragile X anomaly among autistic twins and singletons. *J Child Psychiat.* 1993;34:673-688.

[45] Rutter M, et al. Autism and known medical conditions: myth and substance. *J Child Psychol. Psychiat.* 1994;35:311-322.

[46] Emphasis added.

[47] Bolton P. Developmental Assessment. *Advances in Psychiatric Treatment.* 2001;7:32-42.

[48] Gillberg C and Coleman M. Autism and medical disorders: a review of the literature. *Dev Med and Child Neurol.* 1996;38:191-202.

[49] Hendry CN. Childhood disintegrative disorder: Should it be considered a distinct diagnosis? *Clinical Psychology Review.* 2000;20:77-90.

[50] Rutter M, et al. Autism and known medical conditions: myth and substance. *J Child Psychol and Psychiat.* 1994;35:311-322.

[51] DeLong RG, Bean C, Brown F. Acquired reversible autistic syndrome in acute encephalopathic illness in children. *Child Neurology.* 1981;38:191-194.

[52] Menkes JH and Sarnat HB. *Child Neurology.* 6th Edition. Philadelphia: Lippincott, Williams and Wilkins, 2000.

[53] Menkes JH and Sarnat HB. *Child Neurology.* 6th Edition. Philadelphia: Lippincott, Williams and Wilkins, 2000.

[54] Kinsbourne to Wakefield and Radcliffes Lebrasseur. E-mail. July 2006.

[55] http://62.189.42.105/report/volume1/toc.htm. (no longer available).

[56] Oliveira G, Diogo L, Garcia MP, Miguel ACT, Borges L, Vicente AM, Oliveira CR Mitochondrial dysfunction in autism spectrum disorders: a population-based study. *Developmental Medicine & Child Neurology.* 2005;47:185-189.
Weissman J, Kelley RI, Bauman M, Cohen BH, Murray KF, Mitchell RL, Kern RL. Natowicz MR. Mitochondrial disease in autism spectrum disorder patients: a cohort analysis. PLoS ONE. 2008;3(11):e3815. Doi:101371/journal.pone.0003815
Autism Speaks. (2010) Mitochondria and Autism: Energizing the Study of Energetics. Retrieved from http://www.autismspeaks.org/science/science_news/mitochondria_autism_energetics.php

[57] Bradstreet JJ, El Dahr J, Anthony A, Kartzinel JJ, Wakefield AJ. Detection of Measles Virus Genomic RNA in Cerebrospinal Fluid of Three Children with Regressive Autism: a Report of Three Cases. *Journal of American Physicians and Surgeons.* 2004; 9:38-45 [All children had received MMR and none had a history of measles.]

[58] Statement and report of Professor S. Bustin in UK MMR litigation.

[59] Hornig M, Briese T, Buie T, Bauman ML, Lauwers G, Siemetzki U, Hummel K, Rota PA, Bellini BJ, O'Leary JJ, Sheils O, Alden E, Pickering L, Lipkin WI. Lack of Association between Measles Virus Vaccine and Autism with Enteropathy: A Case-Control Study. *PLoS ONE.* 2008; 3(9):e3140.

[60] Bradstreet JJ, El Dahr J, Montgomery SM, Wakefield AJ. TaqMan RT-PCR Detection of Measles Virus Genomic RNA in Cerebrospinal Fluid in Children with Regressive Autism. Paper presented at International Meeting for Autism Research; Sacramento, California; 2004. [All children had received MMR and none had a history of measles.]

[61] Emphasis added.

[62] American Psychiatric Association. (2009, December 10). *DSM-5 Publication Date Moved to May 2013.* [News Release]. Retrieved from http://www.dsm5.org/Newsroom/Documents/09-65%20DSM%20Timeline.pdf

[63] Gillberg C. Medical Work-Up in Children with Autism and Asperger Syndrome. *Brain Dysfunction.* 1990;3:249-260.

[64] Rutter M, et al. Autism and known medical conditions: myth and substance. *J Child Psychol and Psychiat.* 1994;35:311-322.

[65] United States Court of Federal Claims. King vs Health and Human Services. Case 1:03-vv-00584-UNJ Document 80 Filed 07/01/2008.

[66] Kanner L. Autistic disturbances of affective contact. *Nerv Child.* 1943;2:217-250.

[67] Dohan FC. Schizophrenia: Possible relationship to cereal grains and celiac disease. In: Sankar S, ed. *Schizophrenia: Current Concepts and Research.* Hicksville, NY: PJD Publications, 1968
Goodwin MS, Cowen MA, Goodwin TC., Malabsorption and cerebral dysfunction: a multivariate and comparative study of autistic children, *J Aut Child Schizophr* 1971;1:48-62

[68] Walker-Smith J, Andrews J. Alpha-1-antitrypsin, autism, and coeliac disease. *The Lancet.* 1972;2:883–884.

[69] Gillberg C and Coleman M. *The Biology of the Autistic Syndromes.* New York: Praeger Publications, 1985.

[70] GMC vs Wakefield, Walker-Smith and Murch. Rutter Testimony Tr.38 page 47.

[71] GMC vs Wakefield, Walker-Smith and Murch. Rutter Testimony Tr. 38, page 53.

[72] Krigsman A, Boris M, Goldblatt A, Stott C. Clinical Presentation and Histologic Findings at Ileocolonoscopy in Children with Autistic Spectrum Disorder and Chronic Gastrointestinal Symptoms. *Autism Insights.* 2009;1:1–11.

Horvath K, Perman JA. Autistic disorder and gastrointestinal disease. *Current Opinion in Pediatrics.* 2002;14:583–587.

Melmed RD, Schneider C, Fabes RA, et al. Metabolic markers and gastrointestinal symptoms in children with autism and related disorders. *J Pediatr Gastroenterol Nutr.* 2000;31:S31–S32.

Horvath K, Papadimitriou JC, Rabsztyn A, Drachenberg C, Tildon JT. Gastrointestinal abnormalities in children with autistic disorder. *J Pediatr.* 1999;135:559-63.

Balzola F, Daniela C, Repici A, Barbon A, Sapino A, Barbera C, Calvo PL, Gandione M,

Rigardetto R, Rizzetto M. Autistic enterocolitis: confirmation of a new inflammatory bowel disease in an Italian cohort of patients. *Gastroenterology.* 2005:128 (Suppl 2);A-303.

Gonzalez L, Lopez K, Martınez M et al. Endoscopic and histological characteristics of the digestive mucosa in autistic children with gastrointestinal symptoms. *Arch. Venezolanos Puericultura Y Pediatria.* 2006;69;19–25.

CHAPTER ELEVEN

Disclosure

I have been accused and ultimately found guilty of professional misconduct for not disclosing in *The Lancet* paper that I was a medical expert involved in assessing the merits of litigation against the manufacturers of MMR on behalf of plaintiff children possibly damaged by this vaccine. Notwithstanding the fact that — long before publication — details of my involvement as an expert in the litigation had been provided to my senior coauthors,[1] the dean of the medical school,[2] and the editor of *The Lancet*,[3] it is a matter of fact that it was not disclosed in the published paper.

The Lancet disclosure rules in 1997 were written in the active voice. They asked that the author(s) determine what they considered to constitute a conflict and to disclose or not accordingly (*subjective* duty). At the time of their referral to the Royal Free, not one of the children reported in *The Lancet* was involved in litigation. Each one of those 12 children was referred to Walker-Smith purely for investigation of their symptoms. The matter of litigation had no bearing on *The Lancet* paper.

Moreover, such a disclosure might have conveyed the wrong impression, i.e., that the children's parents were involved in and motivated by litigation, which, to the extent that I can be certain, was not the case. On the basis of these facts, I made the determination that no such disclosure was required. Notably, Horton wrote an editorial in 1997 in defense of his own failure to disclose an author's financial conflict, citing the dangers of becoming obsessed with disclosure and the potential for this obsession to harm free discussion in science.[4] The caution he expressed is particularly relevant in circumstances where such disclosure might create a misleading impression as it might have done with *The Lancet* paper. His apparent plea in mitigation did not, it seems, extend far beyond his own redemption.

Since the early part of the 21st century, disclosure rules have changed. They are now written almost exclusively in the passive voice – what others reviewing or reading the particular paper might perceive as an author's possible or actual conflict(s) of interest (*objective* duty). This is an entirely different ball game. The author is required to put himself in the collective shoes of all potential readers and to disclose anything that he believes they might possibly consider to be a conflict. In the interests of transparency this is commendable, but it is a very different situation as compared with the rules that guided authors in 1998.

What have been the practical consequences for this move to stricter disclosure requirements from 1998 to 2007 for *The Lancet*? For the more than 1000 consecutive contributions written by 3567 authors in volume 351 (January 1 through May 31, 1998), there were declarations of conflicts of interest from only five authors, and these were confined to just two letters. In contrast, performing this same exercise on just two issues of the journal from 2007 (volume 369, number 9579, and volume 370, number 9584), although these contain only 61 consecutive contributions written by 203 authors, there are disclosures of conflicts of interest from 40 authors in 13 articles. With the stricter rules in place, between 1998 and 2007 the rate of disclosures per *Lancet* article went from one in two hundred to more than one in two articles.[5]

Interestingly, while I followed the disclosure rules in 1997 when the paper was submitted to *The Lancet*, at the GMC I was judged according to the current rules. The main reasons for this were twofold, being the evidence of *The Lancet* editor (covered in Chapter 8, "Horton's Evidence") and the opinion of the prosecution's expert witness Professor Sir Michael Rutter. It is upon the latter that I wish to dwell for the remainder of this essay.

Rutter's résumé is impressive, boasting membership on editorial and advisory boards of no fewer than 21 medical journals and over 400 publications in the field of child psychiatry. As an expert witness for the prosecution — paid by the GMC — Rutter enlightened the GMC Panel on the fact that he had been a member of his hospital's ethics committee "for a long time," and, therefore, was an "expert" in conflicts disclosure.[6] He also explained that he was an expert witness on behalf of the vaccine industry in the UK MMR litigation and that he had examined two of *The Lancet 12* children.[7] His opinion on the matter of disclosure inevitably carried considerable weight in the panel's determination of my guilt for lack of disclosure in *The Lancet*.

In his report to the GMC on this matter prior to the hearing, he declared that failure to disclose in *The Lancet* was "quite unsatisfactory."[8] When it came to the hearing, he was considerably more forthright. It is unsettling, therefore, that in his authoritative evidence to the GMC he misrepresented *The Lancet's* standard at the material time.

Smith [Prosecution Counsel]: ...In 1996 if you were a research doctor formulating a research project and subsequently when you submit it for publication, would any possible conflict of interest and I underline we are in 1996 would it be a subject to which you would have given consideration?

*Rutter: Yes, it would be routine to have done so and it is in terms not of the individual investigator's actual conflict of interest as they think but of **perceptions**.[9] There are umpteen documents on ethical issues and they all make clear that it is **perceived conflicts**[9] which are important, and that in 1996 as well as now that would have to be seen as potentially relevant in that it would have to be made explicit.*

Despite *The Lancet's* subjective standard at the material time, Rutter was of the opinion that, then and now, a researcher had an objective duty to disclose conflicting interests. His reason for the disclosure obligation was so that

...the reader of the published research could judge for himself whether the quality of the reported science outweighs the potential for the conflict to bias the interpretation.[10]

While this is laudable, it was not *The Lancet* standard at the material time. At the GMC, Rutter was asked to expand upon the reasoning behind his opinion.

Smith: I know this is a huge subject but you say it would be something in 1996 that should have been given consideration to. Just in broad terms first, what is its relevance to scientific research, why is it regarded as something that should be considered and declared if there is a possible perception?

*Rutter: Because there is actually a [vast] substantial research literature which shows that everybody, that is all of us as well as the rest of the world outside, whether we like it or not, is influenced in our judgments by what we think might be the case, so if there is a reason for favouring one interpretation than another you have to assume that although you may not be conscious of it, it will do so. That is the reason why these things have to be made transparent, made overt, so that people can judge for themselves is the science of such high quality that really the **perceived**[11] possible conflict of interest can be* *cast aside because the evidence is so strong or is this open to a variety of interpretations where the fact that one answer will lead to one sort of outcome and another to a different sort of outcome may influence judgment.*

Once again, Rutter cites an objective standard while *The Lancet* policy on disclosure in 1998 was very narrow and based entirely on the subjective state of mind of the author. The disclosure obligation was subsequently — and appropriately — made much broader and based on an objective third-party standard of what a reasonable person would perceive to be a conflicting interest at *The Lancet* and throughout scientific and medical publishing. However, Rutter faulted me for violating the stricter objective standard well before it was implemented at *The Lancet*.[12] Smith then asked Rutter whether, in theory, *he* would have disclosed *his* involvement in the MMR litigation under the then-applicable standard:

Smith: *...I want to ask you this; putting yourself in the shoes of a reasonably responsible and experienced submitter to medical journals would you regard that test as triggering disclosure in relation to Dr Wakefield's involvement in the litigation?*

Rutter: *Yes, I would, for the reasons I have already given.*

Smith: *Would you regard it as a matter about which a doctor should have any hesitation?*

Rutter: *No hesitation I would have thought.*

Rutter's role in vaccine litigation
As referred to above, Rutter was a paid expert in at least three separate litigation projects on behalf of the vaccine manufacturers and US government; in these projects, he was to offer an expert opinion that thimerosal-containing vaccines and MMR do not cause autism and that the dramatic increase in the incidence of autism is unlikely to be real[13] but simply the result of better ascertainment and a broadening of the diagnostic criteria.

Rutter served as a defendants' expert in US litigation where the plaintiffs alleged that mercury (thimerosal) in vaccines caused autism. He also served as a defendants' expert in the UK MMR litigation which, coincidentally, included two of the children described in *The Lancet* case series. Finally, he was an expert for the US government (in a special vaccine court created by statute in 1986) in the Omnibus Autism Proceeding. He was paid in each of these litigations on the basis of his opinion that vaccines (that is, MMR and/or mercury-containing vaccines) do not cause autism.[14,15]

Rutter offered a similar opinion in an expert report he filed on February 18, 2008, in the US Omnibus Autism Proceeding. His expert opinion, for which he was being well paid, was based in part on his published research.[16] He went on to explain his past and present involvement in litigation.[17]

Rutter was hired to offer his interpretation of the epidemiological data relating to MMR and autism – currently a matter of extensive controversy, debate, and extensive calls for further investigations. Thus, it could be argued that he had and continues to have a financial interest in preserving the absence of evidence in the published medical literature – including his own, much of which he cites in references and footnotes in his expert reports. It is, therefore, the *potential*, if not the *reality*, of his ability to profit substantially from an absence of evidence of causal association in the literature that triggers his obligation to disclose his role as an industry expert in the papers he publishes.

Do as I say, not as I do

But does Rutter do as Rutter says – and not in the laxer, subjective era of the late 1990s, but in the pious, objective era of 2005 and beyond when much stricter rules have applied? Between 2005 and 2008, Rutter published at least five papers in peer-reviewed medical journals that had a direct bearing on the issue of MMR vaccine and autism; for example, these papers include the following statements:

> *The significance of this finding is that MR vaccination is most unlikely to be a main cause of autism.*[18]

> *However, the epidemiological evidence on the main hypothesized environmental explanation, namely the measles-mumps-rubella vaccine, is consistently negative.*[19]

> *There is no support for the hypothesis for a role of either MMR or thimerosal in causation [of autism], but the evidence for the latter is more limited.*[20]

> *The measles-mumps-rubella vaccine was postulated as a risk factor but the epidemiological evidence has been consistently negative.*[21]

With undisguised contempt for those continuing to investigate the potential role of vaccines in autism, this article concludes:

> *There is no disgrace in being wrong, but there is a disgrace in persisting with a theory when empirical findings have made it apparent that the hypothesis or claim was mistaken.*[21]

> *The claims that the so-called "epidemic" of autism was due to either measles-mumps-rubella (MMR) vaccine or the mercury-containing preservative thimerosal that used to be present in many vaccines are not supported by the evidence.*[22]

Nowhere in any of these papers is a disclosure of the fact that Rutter was in the pay of the vaccine manufacturers and the US government to defend their position in vaccine-autism litigation nor is there any disclosure of his role as a paid expert at the GMC. The lack of disclosure in these papers may have occurred for one of two reasons: either Rutter failed to tell the journals' editors, or he did disclose and the editors deemed it unnecessary to avail their readers of this important information, preventing those readers from being able, as Rutter stresses, to "judge for themselves." Only one of the journals makes any mention of disclosure, shedding some light on which of these two alternatives is likely to be correct. At the bottom of Rutter's 2009 article[20] it states:

Conflicts of interest: None declared.

The importance of this matter goes far beyond a simple failure to disclose. In 2005, Rutter was actually on the editorial board of one of the relevant journals, the *Journal of Child Psychology and Psychiatry*, whose position on disclosure – presumably endorsed by Rutter in his editorial role – was very clear.[23]

> *In psychology, as in other scientific disciplines, professional communications are presumed to be based on objective interpretation of evidence and unbiased interpretations of fact. An author's economic and commercial interests in products or services used or discussed in their papers may color such objectivity. Although such relationships do not necessarily constitute a conflict of interest, the integrity of the field requires disclosure of the possibility of such potentially distorting influences where they may exist. The **reader**[24] may then judge and, if necessary, make allowance for the impact of the bias on the information being reported.*

In general, the safest and most open course is to disclose activities and relationships that, if known to others, might be viewed as a conflict of interest, even if you do not believe that any conflict or bias exists.

So, in the interests of transparency, the journal appears to publish disclosures and let the reader decide, indicating that in this instance it was Rutter who failed to disclose. As a paid expert witness for the vaccine industry, Rutter's obligation to disclose was set even higher in 2001 in a commentary[25] published by several editors, including Horton, because, as they explained, such relationships carry a great risk for inappropriate influence and bias.

*Financial relationships (such as employment, consultancies, stock ownership, honoraria, **paid expert testimony**[26]) are the most easily identifiable conflicts of interest and the most likely to undermine the credibility of the journal, the authors, and of science itself... Disclosure of these relationships is particularly important in connection with editorials and review articles, because bias can be more difficult to detect in those publications than in reports of original research.*

Four of Rutter's articles that are cited above fall under the category of "Reviews."

In terms of the significance of Rutter's testimony, his critical role in defining the GMC's position on disclosure and my "dishonesty" was driven home by Smith – erroneously on many levels – on Day 138 of the hearing as she demanded the erasure of my medical license.

The children described in the Lancet paper were... admitted for research purposes under a programme of investigations for Project 172-96. The purpose of the project was to investigate the postulated new syndrome following vaccination. When they were subsequently described in the Lancet paper... Dr Wakefield failed to state that this was the case and that his failure was dishonest, i.e., that he intended to do it and it was irresponsible, and that it resulted in a misleading description of the patient population, a matter which you will recall is fundamental to any scientific paper.

Professor Rutter described it, you will remember, as "absolutely crucial" (Day 37-44E-G). It is fundamental to the readership's understanding of a matter which, in the case of this paper (the Lancet paper) Dr Wakefield knew, as he has admitted, had major public health implications with regard to the public attitude to vaccination, and which he knew would receive a media coverage that would result in nation-wide concern. It is submitted, again, that this is plainly a very grave matter.

Rutter and the GMC

The GMC's ethical guidance for doctors in this case, which is posted as "Acting As An Expert Witness – Guidance for Doctors," requires that an expert witness give honest testimony:[28]

> If you are asked to give evidence or act as a witness in litigation or formal inquiries, you must be honest in all your spoken and written statements. You must make clear the limits of your knowledge or competence.

The ethical guidance amplifies on this requirement by requiring that the expert be "not misleading" and that he "not deliberately leave out relevant information." Finally, the ethical guidance requires that an expert "must be honest, trustworthy, objective, and impartial."

James Moody, Esq., an attorney acting pro bono on behalf of several autism organizations, has written to Rutter, bringing to his attention the fact that these instances of lack of disclosure are to be put in the public domain and offering him the right of reply. The e-mail was sent on March 6, 2010, and a response was requested by March 12, 2010. The respective journal editors have also been contacted. At the time of going to press – April 28, 2010 – no reply has been received.

Rutter is also the subject of a complaint to the GMC claiming that he gave dishonest and misleading expert testimony in violation of the above-cited GMC guidance. As noted above, Rutter has been a paid expert for industry in at least three litigation projects in the UK and US, yet he routinely fails to disclose this conflicting interest in his published papers. Thus, putting himself "in the shoes of a reasonably responsible and experienced submitter to medical journals," as Smith instructed, Rutter could not honestly and in good faith testify that I should have made disclosures – even under the current broader objective standard – because he fails to make the very same disclosures in his own publishing activities.[29] In the light of these facts, the question now is whether he will bring this new evidence to the attention of the GMC.

Based upon the documentary evidence, one is entitled to believe that Rutter uses his position of prominence in the scientific community to publish articles denying any vaccine-autism connection without disclosing his conflicting interest that he was paid by industry lawyers and by the US government (in a statutory program to defend industry in vaccine court) for that very same opinion. While Professor Rutter may well believe his published opinions are independent and honest, the objective standards applicable since approximately 2002 to disclosable conflicts of interest[30] imposed a duty to disclose in published research papers that he was being employed by industry and government to support their position in litigation.

The purpose of this chapter is not to mitigate my lack of disclosure in 1998. I followed the rules and not once did my co-defendants, my boss, or the dean of the medical school – all of whom were aware of my role as an expert in the MMR litigation – ever suggest during the preparation and submission of *The Lancet* paper that disclosure would be appropriate. The merits of this position on disclosure are debatable and this debate – on a matter of opinion – would have been more appropriately held between scientists rather than in the adversarial and punitive arena of a GMC hearing. Rather, this essay is about what amounts to, in my opinion, hypocrisy, double-standards, and professional retribution dressed in sanctimonious piety.

Endnotes

[1] Correspondence between AJW, John-Walker Smith and Simon Murch. February 1997.

[2] Correspondence between AJW and Arie Zuckerman 1996-97.

[3] Correspondence between Richard Barr and Richard Horton. April-July 1997 [see Chapter 8, Horton's Evidence].

[4] Horton R. Conflicts of interest in clinical research: opprobrium or obsession. *The Lancet.* 1997;349:426.

[5] Literature review courtesy of Richard Barr and Kirsten Limb. August 2007.

[6] GMC vs Wakefield, Walker-Smith and Murch. Tr. 35-2C

[7] GMC vs Wakefield, Walker-Smith and Murch. Tr. 35-5B.

[8] GMC vs Wakefield, Walker-Smith Report of Professor Rutter to GMC. p32. 15 may 2007.

[9] Emphasis added.

[10] GMC vs Wakefield, Walker-Smith and Murch. Tr. 37-55D.

[11] Emphasis added.

[12] GMC vs Wakefield, Walker-Smith and Murch. Tr. 37-57C (Ex. 60) (emphasis added)

[13] A real increase would be suggestive of an environmental cause (non-genetic), e.g., vaccines.

[14] Rutter's expert reports have not been made public, but he did testify in US vaccine court on May 27, 2008, in the test cases (Mead and King) In Re: Claims for Vaccine Injuries Resulting in Autism Spectrum Disorders or a Similar Developmental Disorder.

[15] In one expert report in the UK MMR litigation, for example, Professor Rutter offered the opinion in an expert report dated June 23, 2003: "The epidemiological findings show no systematic connection between the timing of the introduction of MMR and the timing of the rise in the rate of autism and other pervasive developmental disorders. Accordingly, the epidemiological findings provide no grounds for concluding that [Child's] disorder is likely to have been associated with MMR."

[16] "With respect to the possibility that toxins may contribute to the causation of mental disorders, I have reviewed the evidence on the effects of environmental lead[5,6,] and have done the same for the effects of the measles-mumps-rubella vaccine[7]. I have published extensively on genetics of mental disorders (Rutter, 2006[8]) and especially on the interplay between genetic and environmental factors (Rutter, 2007[9]; Rutter, in press[10])... With respect to the Vaccine Court hearings, I have particular expertise in the steps needed to identify environmental causes of disease (Academy of Medical Sciences[11], Rutter, 2007[12])... I base my opinions on the available scientific evidence and, in the body of the report, I note the scientific papers that are relevant in relation to individual points. In addition, I also make use of my extensive clinical experience over

the last four decades in diagnosing autism spectrum disorders and treating children and adults with these disorders." [Internal footnotes in original.]

[17] "With respect to the issues being considered by the Vaccine Court, I wish to make explicit that some four years ago I agreed to serve as an expert witness with respect to Thimerosal vaccine litigation. In that connection, I partially drafted a report that, in the event, was never submitted because the litigation was put on hold. Similarly, about a year before that, the same situation arose with respect to litigation over MMR. Once more, the draft report was never finalized and was never submitted because the litigation was dropped. Finally, last year I served as an expert in relation to the British General Medical Council's case against 3 pediatricians involved in Andrew Wakefield's research into autism and MMR. The issues involved there did not concern the scientific case at all but, rather, were involved strictly with the ethical conduct of the research undertaken... Regarding potential conflicts of interest, I declare that throughout the whole of my career I have never received any funding for my research from pharmaceutical companies or any other commercial organization. I agreed to serve as an expert witness in litigation in the UK regarding the mumps – measles – rubella vaccine and received standard fees for the time spent in preparing for this role, but the litigation never resulted in a court hearing."

[18] Honda H, Shimizu Y, Rutter M. No effect of MMR withdrawal on the incidence of autism: a total population study. *Journal of Child Psychology and Psychiatry.* 2005;46:572-579

[19] Rutter M. Aetiology of Autism: Findings and Questions. *J Intellect Disabil Res.* 2005;49(Pt 4):2318.

[20] Rutter M. Incidence of autism spectrum disorders: changes over time and their meaning. *Acta Paediatrica.* 2005;94:2-15.

[21] Rutter M. Autism research: lessons from the past and prospects for the future. *J Autism Dev Disord.* 2005;35:241-257.

[22] Rutter M. Commentary: fact and artifact in the secular increase in the rate of autism. *Int. J. Epidemiol.* 2009;38:1238-1239.

[23] *Journal of Child Psychology and Psychiatry.* Notes for contributors. All authors submitting a paper must complete a Full Disclosure of Interests form. www.apa.org/journals.

[24] Emphasis added.

[25] Davidoff M, et al. Sponsorship, Authorship, and Accountability. *The Lancet.* 2001;358:854 6. This standard was subsequently incorporated into the ICMJE Uniform Requirements for Manuscripts Submitted to Biomedical Journals: Ethical Considerations in the Conduct and Reporting of Research: Conflicts of Interest. See: http://www.icmje.org/ethical_4conflicts.html.

[26] Emphasis added.

[27] GMC vs Wakefield, Walker-Smith, and Murch. Tr. 138

[28] Good Medical Practice: Writing reports and CVs, giving evidence and signing documents. Retrieved from: http://www.gmc-uk.org/guidance/good_medical_practice/probity_reports_and_cvs.asp

[29] GMC vs Wakefield, Walker-Smith and Murch. Tr. 37-57D.

[30] Acting as an expert witness – guidance for doctors. Retrieved from: http://www.gmc-uk.org/guidance/ethical_guidance/expert_witness_guidance.as

CHAPTER TWELVE

Deer

Relations between BD [Brian Deer] and the Sunday Times are at the best of times volatile and there wasn't a story we published in the Sunday Times which wasn't heavily rewritten or cut back.[1]

It may surprise readers who have endured so far that I don't wish to spend any more time than is absolutely necessary on Brian Deer. Despite my wish, this chapter is heavy going. Other chapters deal directly and indirectly with the majority of his original allegations. However, in order to put his journalistic style and quirky perception of events at the Royal Free into context, I will provide a factual analysis of an article he wrote more recently, in fact, at the conclusion of the evidence in the GMC hearing. The article is particularly misleading; clearly a judgment has been made that I represent zero risk as far as defamation goes. When that happens, people can get careless. My sense is that Deer's article was written in some desperation, following a lackluster performance by the prosecution and what appeared to be – at least to many of those in the chamber – a demolition of the GMC's case.

On February 8, 2009, Deer's byline accompanied two related articles in *The Sunday Times*, the first of which was titled

"MMR doctor Andrew Wakefield fixed data on autism."

Blocked excerpts of Deer's articles are provided with a gray background. His articles contained allegations that I committed scientific fraud inasmuch that, apparently, I had "changed and misreported results in [my] research"[2] in *The Lancet* paper, with the clear implication that this was intended to create the appearance of a possible link between MMR vaccination and autism – and that I did it for money.

Since Deer sat through the majority of the GMC hearing where these matters had been aired in considerable detail, he knew or should have known that these allegations were false, misleading, or based on incomplete records and, at the very least, open to question.

The doctor who sparked the scare over the safety of the MMR vaccine for children changed and misreported results in his research, creating the appearance of a possible link with autism, a Sunday Times investigation has found… Confidential medical documents and interviews with witnesses have established that Andrew Wakefield manipulated patients' data, which triggered fears that the MMR triple vaccine to protect against measles, mumps and rubella was linked to the condition.

False: There is no basis in fact for any suggestion that I "manipulated patients' data" at any time. At the GMC, no charge of manipulation or falsification of patient data was brought against me, and none of the evidence presented during the GMC hearing over the year and a half that it took supports any allegation of manipulation of data by me or any of the other 12 coauthors on the paper. The specifics of this allegation are dealt with below.

The research was published in February 1998 in an article in The Lancet medical journal. It claimed that the families of eight out of 12 children attending a routine clinic at the hospital had blamed MMR for their autism, and said that problems came on within days of the jab.

What this clinical paper actually states is that

Onset of behavioural symptoms was associated, by the parents with measles, mumps, and rubella vaccination in eight of the 12 children…

The team also claimed to have discovered a new inflammatory bowel disease underlying the children's conditions.

False: nowhere in *The Lancet* paper is such a claim made.

However, our investigation, confirmed by evidence presented to the General Medical Council (GMC), reveals that: In most of the 12 cases, the children's ailments as described in The Lancet were different from their hospital and GP records.

The documents relevant to the evidence presented in *The Lancet* paper are clearly identified in it and included the Royal Free Hospital (RFH) records and, where available, the developmental records from parents, health visitors [UK registered nurses who visit the home] and GPs. Therefore, as stated in the paper, the team relied on the totality of the information available to us. This is entirely normal practice.

In contrast, the records that were available to the GMC included a complete set of the children's local hospital records, a full set of the GP records including all GPs who had been involved in each child's care, the RFH records, and any other records relating to each child (e.g. school medical records).

Therefore, reliance by Deer upon any differences between these data sources (i.e., those relied on by *The Lancet* authors vis-a-vis those relied upon by Deer in his allegations) is disingenuous and misleading since the majority of the latter records were not available to the Royal Free doctors at the material time.

That is not to say, however, that Deer's interpretation of any differences is accurate. Rather he appears to have cherry-picked differences between these documents with a view to undermining the credibility of *The Lancet* paper. Specific instances of this are provided below.

> *Although the research paper claimed that problems came on within days of the jab, in only one case did medical records suggest this was true, and in many of the cases medical concerns had been raised before the children were vaccinated.*

Labeling our *clinical case series* as a "research paper" is intended to convey the impression that the children were investigated purely for the purposes of experimentation, an allegation that formed a central part of Deer's original complaint to the GMC[3] (see the Afterword, "Ethics, Evidence and the Death of Medicine"). In contrast, the paper reported on the findings in clinically referred children who were investigated on the basis of their presenting symptoms.

> *...that problems came on within days of the jab, in only one case did medical records suggest this was true. In many of the cases medical concerns had been raised before the children were vaccinated.*

False: Deer disingenuously conflates "problems" with "medical concerns." With respect to "problems," *The Lancet* paper was quite specific in referring to the timing of onset of "behavioural problems" in relation to MMR exposure. Nowhere in the paper was any reference was made to the onset of "medical concerns." The latter is an entirely nonspecific expression that might relate to anything that caused a child to present to a doctor. The use of this term to reflect what had been said in *The Lancet* is entirely misleading.

The paper described parental reports of the onset of "behavioural problems" coming on within an average (mean) of 6.5 days after the vaccine. As will be shown below, Deer's implication that these children were exhibiting signs of autism before vaccination is, once again, false or misleading.

Hospital pathologists, looking for inflammatory bowel disease, reported in the majority of cases that the gut was normal. This was then reviewed and the Lancet paper showed them as abnormal.

This allegation illustrates how rigorous clinical and scientific investigation is vulnerable to misrepresentation as a falsification of data. As an example of the fallacy of this allegation, a detailed explanation is provided of the process by which the pathology in tissue biopsies from these children was diagnosed and reported. Firstly, I played no part in the *diagnostic* process at all. Secondly, the fact that a review of the samples took place is clearly spelled out for all to read in *The Lancet* paper itself (see below). There was no sinister attempt to hide any initial assessments as Deer implied.

Biopsies were initially reviewed by duty pathologists who often had no specialist expertise in gastrointestinal disease, particularly in children. Walker-Smith, the senior clinician, who has unparalleled experience of assessing the appearances of bowel disease in children, reviewed all biopsies at a weekly clinicopathological meeting of his team. This was undertaken with the assistance of histopathologist Dr. Sue Davies. At these meetings, Walker-Smith pointed out the fact that inflammation had been overlooked in some of the autism cases.

It was decided that, in order to standardize the analysis of the biopsies, the senior histopathologist with the most expertise in intestinal disease, Dr. Paul Dhillon, should review all biopsies from autistic children. In turn, Dhillon decided that pathology should be graded on a reporting form designed by him[5] to document the presence and severity of microscopic damage. Thereafter, a regular review of biopsies took place involving Drs. Dhillon and Anthony, a trainee pathologist. I was also in attendance. Dhillon's diagnosis formed the basis for what was reported in *The Lancet*. This process has, in fact, been described in the relevant medical literature[1,6] (see below) and was also presented in evidence by me in Deer's presence at the GMC hearing (see below). Once the paper had been written in draft form by me to include Dhillon and Anthony's findings, it was circulated to *all* authors for their modification and approval. Deer should have been aware of these facts before he published his claims; he sat through the evidence, and the details are set out in the published literature.

Documented below and available to Deer at the time of writing his article are the specific references to this diagnostic process, which appeared in *The Lancet* 1998 paper and two subsequent published papers in 2000 and 2004.

Ileal lymphoid nodular hyperplasia, non-specific colitis, and pervasive developmental disorder in children[7]

Formalin-fixed biopsy samples from ileum and colon were assessed and reported by a pathologist (SED).[8] Five ileocolonic biopsy series from age-matched and site-matched controls whose reports showed histologically normal mucosa were obtained for comparison. All tissues were assessed by three other clinical and experimental pathologists (APD, AA, AJW).[9]

This process was reported in greater detail in follow-up studies that included the 12 *Lancet* children.[10] The Results section of this same paper documented a high degree of agreement between independent pathologists in an observer-blinded analysis (i.e., where the person scoring the biopsy was unaware of the diagnosis in the individual from whom the biopsy came and the score given to the same biopsy by other observers).[11]

A further publication provided a detailed review of the diagnostic process, specifically referring to the roles of Dhillon and Anthony. It also referred to the clinicopathological meeting and the fact that pathological findings were frequently modified as a consequence of this expert and thorough review process.[12] The details of the diagnostic process were also described by me during evidence (Days 49 and 50) at the GMC with Deer in attendance.[13]

Dhillon's role in the diagnostic process is *also* confirmed in a statement he provided to the GMC and that was signed by him on July 28, 2006.[14] This key document confirms his role in making the diagnosis in *The Lancet* children in the most stringent way, i.e., by a *blinded review* as described above.

There should have been no doubt in anyone's mind at the GMC hearing as to the extraordinary diligence with which the diagnostic process was carried out and the fact that I was not in any way responsible for the final tissue diagnosis in *The Lancet* children.

Back to Deer…

> *Through his lawyers, Wakefield this weekend denied the issues raised by our investigation, but declined to comment further.*

Unfortunately, Deer's allegations were only provided to me on the morning of Friday, February 6, 2009. I was given a deadline of Saturday, February 7, midday London time, i.e., 6:00 A.M. Central Standard Time in Texas, leaving no adequate time for me or my legal team to deal with the matter.

The following section deals with the accompanying story on the inside pages that appeared in *The Sunday Times* of February 8, 2009. It is concerned with specific allegations with respect to individual children.

Hidden records show MMR truth

A Sunday Times investigation has found that altered data was behind the decade-long scare over vaccination.

Its research caused one of the biggest stirs in modern medical history when its results were published in The Lancet medical journal. The five-page paper suggested a potential link between MMR and what the doctors called a "syndrome" of autism and inflammatory bowel disease.

The children were not named in the tables of results. Eleven boys and one girl, aged between 2½ and 9½, were said, for the most part, to have a diagnosis of regressive autism, where children appear to develop quite normally, but then, terrifyingly, lose their language skills. The bowel disease was described as nonspecific colitis, a severe form of inflammation.

The dynamite in The Lancet was the claim that their conditions could be linked to the MMR vaccine, which had been given to all 12 children.

False: *The Lancet* paper did not "claim that their conditions could be linked to the MMR vaccine." No such claim was ever made in the paper; on the contrary, it was explicitly stated in that paper that *no association* – let alone a causal association – had been proved between MMR and the syndrome described. It reported only that the parents said onset of symptoms started after MMR vaccination in 8 of 12 cases.

According to the paper, published on February 28, 1998, the parents of eight of the children said their "previously normal" child developed "behavioural symptoms" within days of receiving the jab.

"In these eight children the average interval from exposure to first behavioural symptoms was 6.3 days," said the paper.

At face value, these findings were more than grounds for the panic that took off over MMR. If such startling results were obtained from two-thirds of a group of previously normal children turning up at one clinic at just one hospital, what might be happening, unreported, all over the world? This might be the first snapshot of a hidden catastrophe, a secret epidemic of vaccine damage.

To launch the findings, the Royal Free held a press conference, and issued a video news release. The researchers' leader, Dr Andrew Wakefield, then 41, was emphatic in his comments to the assembled media.

"It's a moral issue for me," he said. "I can't support the continued use of these three vaccines, given in combination, until this issue has been resolved."

Eleven years later, the fallout continues around the world. The paper triggered a public health crisis. In Britain, immunisation rates collapsed from 92% before the Lancet paper was published, to 80% at the peak of Britain's alarm. Measles has returned as officially "endemic".

With less than 95% of the population vaccinated, Britain has lost its herd immunity against the disease. In 1998 there were 56 cases reported; last year there were 1,348, according to figures released last week that showed a 36% increase in 2007. Two British children have died from measles, and others put on ventilators, while many parents of autistic children torture themselves for having let a son or daughter receive the injection.

"There's not a day go by I don't cry because of what happened," said the mother of a severely disabled 12-year-old girl. "I shouldn't have took her [for the MMR], and you know everyone will say, 'Don't blame yourself', but I do. I blame myself."

Yet the science remains a problem. No researchers have been able to replicate the results produced by Wakefield's team in the Lancet study.

False: It was not true to say there had been no replication of the work as stated above; three independent groups have reported on intestinal inflammation (ileitis and colitis) in children with autism since the initial 1998 publication in *The Lancet*.[15] Similar findings of bowel disease have since been published by three groups.[16]

Some used statistics to see if autism took off in 1988, when MMR was introduced. It did not.

False: Although ecological data provide little more than correlations, in the UK autism did take off when MMR vaccine was introduced. A paper from Taylor et al.[17] showed this correlation when crucial factors such as the inclusion of older children who had been part of a *catch up* campaign — omitted from the original paper — were taken into consideration.[18]

Others used virology to see if MMR caused bowel disease, a core suggestion in the paper. It did not.

This claim is misleading and betrays ignorance, an attempt to mislead, or both. Virology has been used for the detection of measles virus and other viruses in the intestinal tissues of children with autism. Whether measles virus is present or not, "virology" tests, as used, cannot "see if MMR caused the bowel disease," it can only determine presence or absence of a particular virus and, at most, indicate a possible association.

Yet more replicated the exact Wakefield tests. They showed nothing like what he said.

False: Firstly, the tests reported in *The Lancet* paper are not in any manner "Wakefield tests," but clinical investigations that were deemed necessary by the appropriate clinicians. No details are provided in support of Deer's claim nor are the assertions attributed to any expert. As shown above, those studies that have looked for bowel disease in autistic children with gastrointestinal symptoms have found it.[15,16]

Wakefield himself, however, stands by his results, insisting that a link between MMR and autism merits inquiry. The 12 other doctors whose names were attached to the Lancet paper, which was written by Wakefield, were not involved in preparing the data used.

False: The other authors generated and, indeed, prepared all the data that was reported in *The Lancet*. I merely put their completed data in tables and narrative form for the purpose of submission for publication. All authors were provided with drafts of the paper for the purpose of checking their data and making amendments as necessary prior to submission.

> *"This study created a sensation among the public that was impossible to counter, despite overwhelming evidence to the contrary," says Professor Gary Freed, director of the child health research unit at the University of Michigan, who has watched the scare take off in America.*
>
> *"Overwhelming biologic and epidemiologic evidence has demonstrated conclusively that there is no association between the MMR vaccine and autism, and yet this thing goes on." Aspects of the project are now before the General Medical Council (GMC), the doctors' disciplinary body.*
>
> *Wakefield and two professors, John Walker-Smith, 72, and Simon Murch, 52, are charged with carrying out unauthorised research on the 12 children. The charges, which they strongly deny, relate to the ethics of the treatment of the 12 children, not the results of the research.*
>
> *In evidence presented to the GMC, however, there has emerged potential explanations of how Wakefield was able to obtain the results he did. This evidence, combined with unprecedented access to medical records, a mass of confidential documents and cooperation from parents during an investigation by this newspaper, has shown the selective reporting and changes to findings that allowed a link between MMR and autism to be asserted.*

Deer's statement is clearly intended to convey the impression that it was I who "obtain[ed] the results" and that these results were obtained by my "selective reporting and changes," with the clear implication of scientific fraud on my part, for the purpose of allowing "a link between MMR and autism to be asserted."

False: I did not *obtain* the results in the sense that is intended. The results were obtained by the clinicians investigating these children. I had no role in obtaining these results other than to collate them for publication. The process by which the clinicians obtained the results is apparent in *The Lancet* paper and had been described in great detail to the GMC hearing.

The only thing that "allowed a link between MMR and autism" to be suggested was the parental history. This was faithfully reported in *The Lancet*.

...at the heart of Wakefield's findings The Sunday Times found more discrepancies, inconsistencies and changes.

Much of the anonymized information which follows comes from the medical records of disabled children – confidential records held by Deer but intended solely for use by clinicians involved in the children's care. Deer's allegations address two aspects: these are the history of the relationship of MMR to the pattern of onset of the children's symptoms and the microscopic examination of the children's intestinal tissues.

It is essential to note that *The Lancet* paper clearly stated that the history of the onset of behavioral symptoms was associated by the parents with MMR in 8 of the 12 children, and it is the initial behavioral symptoms described by the parents that we reported. With respect to the timing of the MMR and the onset of symptoms, Deer relies upon evidence in the children identified as 1, 2, 6, 7 and 8 of *The Lancet 12*.

Child 1

The first, in the Lancet tables, concerned the first child in the paper: Child One, from Cottesmore, Leicestershire. He was 3½ years old and the son of an air force pilot. In November 1995, his parents had been devastated after receiving a diagnosis of autism.

"Mr and Mrs [One]'s most recent concern is that the MMR vaccination given to their son may be responsible," their GP told the hospital in a letter.

In the paper this claim would be adopted, with Wakefield and his team reporting that Child One's parents said "behavioural symptoms" started "one week" after he received the MMR.

Child 1 was reported as suffering "fever and delirium." This delirium started 1 week after MMR vaccination and lasted for 3 days[19] and denotes his first behavioral symptom as specifically stated in *The Lancet*.[20] With respect to his subsequent clinical course, Walker-Smith, in his letter to the GP stated,

Between the age of 1 year and 18 months his development slowed and then deteriorated.[21]

Evidence from Child 1's GP at the GMC hearing confirmed that Mrs. 1's view was that her child had developed normally until he had his MMR vaccine. This was documented in the medical records and formed the basis of the information contained in *The Lancet* paper. The facts are entirely accurate as reported.

> *The boy's medical records reveal a subtly different story, one familiar to mothers and fathers of autistic children. At the age of 9½ months, 10 weeks before his jab, his mother had become worried that he did not hear properly: the classic first symptom presented by sufferers of autism. Child One was among the eight reported with the apparent sudden onset of the condition.*

A review of the additional GP records (not available to the Royal Free team at the time of writing *The Lancet* paper) shows that, with respect to his claim about Child 1's hearing, Deer fails to mention the crucial fact that in the entry documenting his mother's concerns about Child 1's hearing, her additional concern was about a discharge from Child 1's left ear.[22] This concern is not suggestive of an incipient developmental disorder but of an ear infection. This would have been sufficient reason for his mother to express possible concerns about Child 1's hearing. Here we have an example of Deer's highly selective reporting of results that were not available to the authors of *The Lancet* paper at the material time. Throughout his reporting, Deer appears to rely selectively on such "facts" that support his premise that I have perpetrated a fraud.

Child 1's Royal Free Hospital records contain no reference whatsoever to any hearing difficulties. These records include the referral letter from the GP to Professor Walker-Smith. The only reference to Child 1's hearing is in the Royal Free Hospital record of January 21, 1996, where his hearing is reported as being "normal."[23]

The health visitor records[24] were available to the Royal Free team and are described below.

"11.3.93 Hearing and development normal."[25]

"12.8.93 Hearing and development normal."[26]

Child 2

> *So was the next child to be admitted. This was Child Two, an eight-year-old boy from Peterborough, Cambridgeshire, diagnosed with regressive autism, which, according to the Lancet paper, started "two weeks" after his jab.*
>
> *However, this child's medical records, backed by numerous specialist assessments, said his problems began three to five months later.*

The Lancet paper described the onset of Child 2's first behavioral symptoms as having occurred 2 weeks after MMR vaccination. The first reference to onset of his behavioral symptoms, as correctly reported in *The Lancet*, is found in the assessment of Child 2 by consultant child psychiatrist Dr. Mark Berelowitz in Child 2's Royal Free Hospital records as described in a letter to Dr. Simon Murch:[27]

> [Child 2's] *milestones in the 1st year were normal. At the age of 13 months she* [Child 2's mother] *said he had 25 words, but he gradually lost his words over the next 7 to 8 months. ...his Fragile X was negative his brain scan is normal as is his EEG...*[his mother] *reiterated that* [Child 2] **started head banging about 2 weeks after the MMR and hasn't looked right since.**[28] *I thought that the history and presentation were very typical of autism or a related disorder...*

This is confirmed in the Royal Free records in the discharge summary:

> *Until 20 months of age... normal developmental progress. ... Mum does recount that at 13 months of age he had had his MMR immunisation and 2 weeks following this had started with* <u>head banging behaviour</u> <u>and screaming throughout the night.</u> *He subsequently seemed generally sickly.*[29]

The problem became progressively more severe with loss of language, incoordination, and other features of developmental regression, but the first behavioral symptom was correctly stated as

> *...head banging about 2 weeks after the MMR.*

There are additional references in the Royal Free Hospital records from the senior medical authors of the paper to his subsequent developmental deterioration. These include an outpatient note from Walker-Smith that said "*had MMR at 15 months* [This is an error by JWS that should read '13 months'], *went down hill ever since.*"[30] And a letter from Berelowitz dated September 30, 1996, said *"had 25 words at 13 months which he then lost, began to get a bit clumsy at 15 months."*[31]

> *The difference between 14 days and a few months is significant, according to experts. Autism usually reveals itself in the second year of life, when the vaccine is routinely given. If there was no sudden onset after the MMR injection, as claimed for the "syndrome", the condition could be ascribed to a conventional pattern.*

The sudden onset of Child 2's behavioral symptoms means that his condition could not be ascribed to "a conventional pattern." In fact, elsewhere in his records, not referenced by Deer, experts describe his regressive pattern of autism as "unusual."[32] Deer failed to include this information.

Child 6 and Child 7

> *More apparent anomalies lurked among the following 10 children, as they arrived at the Royal Free hospital between September 1996 and February 1997.*
>
> *Child Six, aged 5, and Child Seven, aged 3, were said to have been diagnosed with regressive autism, with an onset of symptoms "one week" and "24 hours" after the jab respectively.*
>
> *But medical records show that neither boy was "previously normal", as the Lancet article described all the children, and that both had already been hospitalised with brain problems before their MMR.*

False: *The Lancet* article described these two children as having "normal development followed by loss of acquired skills." It did *not* say that they were "previously normal" which is a nonspecific term, potentially covering all aspects of their health. The paper did *not* state that these children had been diagnosed with "regressive autism" as Deer reported. In fact, at the time that paper was written, "regressive autism" was not a recognized diagnosis. Over the years, they were diagnosed with various behavioral labels within the autistic spectrum including autism, Asperger's syndrome, and PDD. The clinical history and the medical records confirm that they underwent developmental regression, having been previously developmentally normal.

Child 6

> *Child Six received his vaccine at the age of 14 months, but had twice previously been admitted with fits.*

Whether or not Child 6 suffered from "fits," this point is irrelevant to the fact that his early development prior to MMR was considered normal. His fit was a febrile convulsion[33] which is not uncommon in children with fever and is certainly not indicative of an underlying brain problem or incipient autism.

Child 6's early development prior to MMR was normal according to documents supplied to the Royal Free.[34]

It is notable that he should not have received MMR vaccine in view of his history of seizures. In a letter to the consultant community pediatrician on May 19, 1997, Child 6's doctor wrote this from the RFH:

> *Mum gave a history in* [Child 6] *of changes in social interaction following on immediately from his MMR vaccination.*[35]

Consistent with the changes in social interaction, Child 6's initial behavioral symptom was confirmed by his mother and was described in *The Lancet* as "gaze avoidance."[36] Thus, Child 6's initial behavioral symptom was accurately reported in *The Lancet*.

Child 7

> *Child Seven was given his MMR at the age of 20 months but, again, problems already showed.*
>
> *"He developed well, had social smiling and was responsive to his mother,"* a psychiatrist wrote. *"But he began to have pale episodes and* [sic] *petit mal* [convulsions]*, and had an EEG* [an electroencephalogram, a common test for epilepsy] *done at 15 months, which was abnormal."*

Once again, *The Lancet* paper specifically reported on the developmental status of children, and Child 7 was developmentally normal prior to his MMR. It is also notable that in view of his history of fits, he should never have received an MMR vaccine.

Health visitor records are available from December 21, 1994, at 10 months of age showing his development as entirely normal with no concerns whatsoever.[37]

There is an entry in his GP's records on September 27, 1995, at 19 months of age that states "happy baby."[38]

In spite of his history of seizures, his developmental trajectory was entirely normal as evidenced by an entry in his GP's records when he was just under 20 months of age: "Development normal."[39]

Child 7 received his MMR at 21 months of age on November 24, 1995.[40] In May 1996, his GP record states:

> ...bowel problems, constipation and bleeding. MMR Nov 95, quieter since, never happy, does not laugh. Cry or whine all day, falling, unsteady.[41]

He continued to deteriorate, and on January 29, 1996, his local hospital records read:

> Significant change in behaviour past 2 weeks. He became aggressive and incontinent.[42]

The change following MMR vaccination is described in a letter dated January 21, 1997, from Walker-Smith to Child 7's GP in response to his referral:

> Many thanks for referring [Child 7]. I was very interested to hear the history of this child in which there does seem to be a clear relationship between symptomatology and the MMR. He had the MMR rather later than the usual at 21 months. His mother tells me that 24 hours afterwards he had a fit-like episode and slept poorly thereafter and she attributes changes in his behaviour to this event.

Let's return to Deer:

> Meanwhile, neither [Child 6 nor Child 7] was diagnosed with regressive autism, or even nonregressive classical autism. Three of the children had been diagnosed with Asperger's disorder, in which language is not lost, and which is not regressive: nothing like what afflicted One and Two. This was also the diagnosis for Child Twelve in the series, a six-year-old boy from Burgess Hill, West Sussex.

Child 6

False: Based upon this child's records he received various diagnoses on the autistic spectrum over the years, including autism[43] and autistic spectrum disorder.[44] Evidence of Child 6's regression can be found at various places in his records.[45] Child 6's GP confirmed the mother's perception of the relationship of Child 6's autism to MMR in his evidence to the GMC on July 20, 2007:

Q: As far as you understood, Doctor, did this child's mother have beliefs as to the reason why Child 6 was autistic?

A: Yes.

Q: Can you tell us what they were and, if you can remember, when she first made them clear to you?

A: I am not sure when she first made them clear, probably from an early stage. She was convinced that it was to do with the MMR vaccination. She said he was fine before then.

And Seven would be diagnosed with an odd behavioural condition called "pathological demand avoidance syndrome" [PDA]. This usually manifests as social manipulativeness, and is nothing like the "syndrome" being claimed. It is sometimes marked by a child putting his hands on his ears, while singing "lah-lah-lah, can't hear you".

Child 7's records confirm that he was developmentally normal prior to MMR.[46] In contrast with the claim that Child 7's clinical course was "nothing like the syndrome being claimed," his history is captured in Walker-Smith's letter of January 21, 1997, to the referring GP as described above. There are many references to Child 7's behavioral and developmental regression in the records.[47] And in contrast with Deer's claim that Child 7 did not have an autism diagnosis, his records show that, as with other children, Child 7's diagnosis changed over time as his condition developed and included not just PDA, but was documented as "autism," and "autistic spectrum disorder."[48]

Child 8

Only one was a girl, Child Eight, aged 3, from Whitley Bay, Tyne & Wear. She was reported in the journal as having suffered a brain injury "two weeks" after MMR.

Her medical records did not support this. Before she was admitted, she had been seen by local specialists, and her GP told the Royal Free of "significant concerns" about her development some months before she had her MMR.

Mrs 8 expressed concerns about 8's health and development from an early stage.

False: Child 8 was reported in *The Lancet* as follows:

The only girl (child number 8) was noted to be a slow developer compared with her older sister.[49] *She was subsequently found to have coarctation of the aorta. After surgical repair of the aorta at 14 months, she progressed rapidly, and learnt to talk. Speech was lost later.*

Based upon the diagnosis of Berelowitz, the Royal Free's child psychiatrist, she is reported in *The Lancet* as having a possible post-vaccine encephalitis (brain inflammation). In contrast with Deer's false assertion, her medical records confirm exactly the history that was reported in *The Lancet*. This report is supported by her records of what Berelowitz interpreted as a likely encephalitic episode.

Within 2 weeks of MMR at 19 months developed rash and febrile convulsions... followed by behavioural deterioration, loss of words and vocalisation, screaming, hyperacusis, ataxia and nocturnal myoclonic jerks.[50]

Berelowitz continued:

MMR Jan 95, grand mal convulsion Feb 95 2 weeks after MMR, never the same again.[51]

The description of Child 8 in *The Lancet* is an entirely accurate representation of her history as documented in her clinical record and described below. In particular, Deer omits the critical fact that because of the concerns of developmental delay, she was assessed twice prior to MMR by a local developmental pediatrician who reported he considered her to be within the normal range for development on both occasions.[52] These assessments took place at the ages of 10.5 months (May 20, 1994) and 17 months (December 16, 1994). In December 1994, her development was considered age appropriate.

Child 8 suffered from coarctation of the aorta. This would readily account for her mother's concerns about her slow development. The mother's concerns about Child 8's development were with reference to her development relative to her sister[53] as reported in *The Lancet*.

Of note is her GP's comment in her referral letter to the Royal Free Hospital of October 3, 1996:

[Child 8's] *development did appear to get worse following the MMR.*[54]

Child 8's GP comments in her statement made to the GMC[55] that Child 8 received her MMR on January 27, 1995, and that since then Mrs. 8 "perceived a definite reversal" in Child 8's development.

What is striking is that in February 1995 (Child 8 seen on February 17; letter dictated March 2, 1995), a matter of weeks after her MMR, she was once again reviewed by the same developmental pediatrician (Dr. Houslby) who now determined that she was "globally developmentally delayed functioning at about the one year level."[56]

Thus, within the space of just 1 month, Child 8 had deteriorated considerably. Rather than progressing developmentally, she had gone from functioning at around the 18-month level down to the 1-year level in 1 month. Very little, if any, attention seems to have been paid to this. Child 8's reaction to the MMR vaccine, although acknowledged, received no further consideration and no appropriate investigation.

There is a great deal of evidence of regression in Child 8's medical history and a clear paper trail of her mother's association of her problems with the MMR, long before any contact with doctors at the Royal Free Hospital. This is corroborated by multiple references in Child 8's records:[57]

During the GMC hearing, Child 8's GP gave the following evidence:[58]

Q: What was the mother of Child 8's perception of Child 8's reaction to the vaccine?

A: I felt that the mother was concerned fairly soon after the vaccine – I think I saw her at home on a home visit shortly after the vaccination – she had had a kind of feverish reaction to it. There obviously was no suggestion of delay at that point. Several months later her mum said she had been looking at a video when Child 8 had a little bit of speech before the vaccination and she felt that that had reduced post-vaccination.

Q: The incident you describe of the video was some time later, was it?

A: Yes.

Q: In terms of the more immediate reaction to the vaccine, you say that mum reported a fever.

A: Yes. I remember seeing her at home and then I think she was admitted with a febrile convulsion shortly afterwards.

A letter from Dr. Bushby, the geneticist, to a GP, Dr. Tapsfield, provided further confirmation of Child 8's reaction to MMR.[59]

In summary, the reporting of Child 8's behavioral and developmental history in *The Lancet* paper was entirely accurate. In contrast, Deer's allegation that her medical records did not support her description in *The Lancet* is false.

Allegations of changing histopathological[60] findings in the children's biopsies
The meticulous process by which the pathology in tissue biopsies from *The Lancet 12* was diagnosed and reported has already been described. With regard to the alleged misrepresentation of the pathology, Deer relies on evidence related to children 3, 8, 9, and 10.

When the children first arrived at the Royal Free, in addition to autism, they were also reported with constipation, diarrhoea or other common bowel complaints. This was the reason given for them travelling between 60 and 5,000 miles to London to enter the care of Wakefield's team.

The Lancet 12 all had gastrointestinal symptoms including abdominal pain, diarrhea, laxative-dependent constipation, bloating, and, in some cases, food intolerance.

It is misleading to suggest that they entered the care of "Wakefield's team." Deer is well aware that all of these children were under the clinical care of John Walker-Smith's team of pediatric gastroenterologists at the Royal Free. At no time were they under the care of "Wakefield's team"— there was no such team offering care to children.

Wakefield, now 52, a former gut surgeon, was at the time doing academic research in the Royal Free's medical school on Crohn's disease, an ulcerating inflammation. In 1995, he had developed a theory that this condition was caused by the measles virus, which is found live in MMR. The theory has since been discounted.

False: The theory has not been discounted.

This work was the bedrock on which he based his new claims. Yet this too appears problematic. The children were supposed to have a

> *new inflammatory bowel disease, written up in the Lancet paper as "consistent gastrointestinal findings" involving "nonspecific colitis". Wakefield said that this inflammation of the colon caused the gut to become "leaky", allowing food-derived poisons to pass into the bloodstream and the brain.*

False: Any new claim was that these children had bowel disease; any relationship between measles virus and Crohn's disease had no bearing on this, let alone forming its "bedrock."

False: *The Lancet* paper did not claim that the children were supposed to have a new inflammatory bowel disease.

False: I did not say that "this inflammation of the colon caused the gut to become 'leaky', allowing food-derived poisons to pass into the bloodstream and the brain." This was merely a hypothesis that was presented as such in the Discussion section of the paper.

> *"The uniformity of the intestinal pathological changes and the fact that previous studies have found intestinal dysfunction in children with autistic-spectrum disorders, suggests that the connection is real and reflects a unique disease process," the Lancet Paper explained of the "syndrome".*
>
> *Yet pathology records of samples taken from the children show apparent problems with this evidence. The hospital's consultants who took biopsies from the children's colons concluded that they were not uniform but varied and unexceptional.*

Let me review for you the claims and what the reports *actually* said.

Child 8

> *For Child Eight, the pathology report said: "No abnormality detected", while the Lancet paper said: "Nonspecific colitis". This pattern was repeated for two [Child 9 and Child 10] of the other children."*

Child 8's routine report, undertaken by a neuropathologist (an expert in brain pathology), in fact described "minimal inflammatory changes."[61] This was confirmed in a letter from Dr. David Casson of November 27, 1997, noting that "All pieces of colonic tissue demonstrated minimal inflammatory changes."[62]

When the biopsies were reviewed and scored by experts in bowel pathology, namely Dhillon and Anthony, these doctors determined that there was mild inflammation in the cecum, ascending colon, and rectum.[63] This was correctly reported as "nonspecific colitis" in *The Lancet.*

Child 9

Child 9's clinical histopathology was reported in the routine pathology laboratory as showing "no histological abnormality."[64] Walker-Smith reviewed Child 9's biopsies directly with Dhillon. Both agreed that the biopsies, in fact, showed inflammation consistent with an indeterminate colitis.[65,66] In addition, the research scoring by Dhillon and Anthony recorded this:

> *Increase in chronic inflammatory cells, cryptitis, reactive follicular hyperplasia, and increase in intraepithelial lymphocytes.*[67]

A revised diagnosis of "indeterminate colitis" was made, which was communicated to the child's doctor by Walker-Smith. This diagnosis was reported in *The Lancet.*

Child 10

Child 10's routine histopathology report was provided by an expert in gynecological pathology. It said the following:

> *No significant histological abnormality*[68]

When reviewed by Walker-Smith's clinical team, it was evident to them that the biopsies showed abnormality, and a supplementary report was requested which described mild chronic inflammation.[69] The biopsies were reviewed by Dhillon and Anthony who reported

> *Mild chronic inflammation in the caecum, ascending, transverse, and sigmoid colon, and rectum.*[70]

This was correctly reported in *The Lancet.*

Child 3

> *The **most striking change of opinion came**[71] in the case of Child Three, a six-year-old from Huyton, Merseyside. He was reported in the journal to be suffering from regressive autism and bowel disease: specifically "acute and chronic nonspecific colitis". The boy's hospital discharge summary, however, said there was nothing untoward in his biopsy.*

False: Child 10's initial routine histopathology report, provided by Dhillon, was abnormal. It read:

Small bowel mucosa shows an increase in intra-epithelial small lymphocytes; and, Mild inflammatory and reactive changes in the small bowel samples.[72]

Following his review, Walker-Smith noted:

Marked increase in IEL's [intra-epithelial lymphocytes] in ileum with chronic inflammatory cells. Increase in inflammatory cells in colon and IEL's increased.[73]

The biopsies were reviewed by Dhillon and Anthony who reported:

Mild chronic inflammation in the caecum, and ascending and sigmoid colon, and rectum, with mild-to-moderate inflammation in the transverse colon.[74]

These findings were communicated by the clinical team to Child 3's GP Dr. Shantha[75] in a letter of April 10, 1996, from Dr. David Casson (a lecturer in pediatric gastroenterology).

Small bowel mucosa showed an increase in intra-epithelial lymphocytes but there was [sic] no architectural abnormalities. Histology of the terminal ileum showed prominent lymphoid follicles. Colonic histology was all reported as within normal histological limits. Overall there appeared to be therefore mild inflammatory reactive changes in the small bowel samples.

In other words, his records show a blatant contradiction between what Deer reported and what is clearly and consistently stated in the clinical records.

Once the biopsies had been reviewed by Walker-Smith's clinical team, the histological findings were revised, and a letter was sent to Child 3's GP informing him of this change and the resulting treatment recommendations. In a letter of December 31, 1996, Walker-Smith wrote to Dr. Shantha:

You remember you kindly referred [Child 3] to me and we sent a discharge summary to you on the 4th of October, 1996. Further critical analysis of histology results have led to an amendment to the discharge summary which I am now enclosing. Our final diagnosis is of indeterminate ileocolitis with lymphonodular hyperplasia. In the light of these histological findings and if gastrointestinal symptoms persist, treatment with a drug such as Asacol might be of some therapeutic value...[76]

The discharge summary was revised by hand by a Dr. Hepstead to read as follows:

Diagnosis: indeterminate ileo-colitis and lymphoid nodular hyperplasia.[77]

Under the histology section, the revision reads:

Ileal mucosa shows an increase in intra-epithelial lymphocytes but there are no architectural abnormalities. Histology of the terminal ileum showed prominent lymphoid follicles. Colonic histology revealed an increase of chronic inflammatory cells.

Motivated by Litigation?

Further questions arise about the motivations of Wakefield. Five years ago this month, The Sunday Times reported that he worked for lawyers, and that many of the families were either litigants or were part of networks through which they would sue. Far from routine referrals, as they appeared, many of them had made contact with one another.

The clear inference from Deer's statement is that the children's referral was motivated by the fact that they were litigants. In fact, at the time of their referral to the Royal Free Hospital none of the children were litigants. Only one child (Child 12) received a legal aid certificate in the interval between his referral to Walker-Smith and his first attendance at the Royal Free. This was captured in my evidence on Day 53 of the GMC hearing.[79]

Child 6 and Child 7

Child Six and Child Seven were brothers from East Sussex; Child Four, a 9½-year-old from North Shields, Tyneside, was registered with the same GP as Child Eight. In short, the 12, none of whom came from London, fetched up far-from-routinely at the hospital.

As stated in *The Lancet*, children were referred by their GPs or pediatricians as is routine practice in the National Health Service. This was a group of children referred to an expert team in a tertiary referral center with a particular expertise in childhood bowel disease for investigation of their intestinal symptoms. Their referral had absolutely nothing to do with litigation,[80] and there has been no evidence produced in support of this claim. In his evidence on Day 73 of the hearing, Walker-Smith confirmed the clinical basis of the children's investigations.[81] Later that same day he was asked whether the children were genuinely ill:

> Q: Did it prove to be the case, that they were seriously sick children?
>
> A: They were. They were in some ways really quite shocking, in the sense that the parents had had a child which was perfectly well and then, quite dramatically, over a short period of time, major behavioural problems and bowel problems had appeared. There was video evidence and photographic evidence of the children before and after in some cases.

There was no such sense of empathy from Deer in *The Sunday Times*.

> The mothers of Child Two and Child Three told me what others said in medical records: they had heard of Wakefield through the MMR vaccine campaign, Jabs. (sic)
>
> Thus, when they arrived on Malcolm ward, and **produced the "finding" about MMR**,[82] it was by no means a random sample of cases.

The Lancet paper described the findings of what was clearly described as a "self-referred group" of patients. It has never been suggested by any of the authors that this was a "random sample of cases."

> What parents did not know was that, two years before, Wakefield had been hired by Jabs's[83] [sic] lawyer, Richard Barr, a high-street solicitor in King's Lynn, Norfolk. Barr had obtained legal aid to probe MMR for any evidence that could be used against the manufacturers.

False: Deer has no knowledge of the parents' state of mind. My role in the MMR litigation was public knowledge from an early stage. For example, *The Independent* newspaper carried a story on November 27, 1996, called "Law: A shot in the Dark."[84] The second paragraph opened with:

> William is one of 10 children taking part in a pilot study at the Royal Free Hospital in London, which is investigating possible links between the measles vaccine with the bowel disorder Crohn's disease, and with autism.

Deer wrote:

> *...There is no suggestion the other doctors knew of Wakefield's involvement with Barr.*

False: My colleagues' state of knowledge is clearly documented in papers that were in Deer's possession and adduced in evidence to the GMC. Specifically, I first wrote to Walker-Smith about a patient in November 1996 informing him that this child had been awarded funding from the LAB that would, if necessary, cover the costs of his investigation.[85] This is clarified in my evidence on Day 53 of the GMC hearing:

> *Q: Can I now leave that background material, and move back to the Royal Free records, page 76. On 6 November you wrote to Professor Walker-Smith about this patient, in these terms:*
>
> *"This is a child that I would like to be included in our study if you consider him suitable. His community paediatrician, Dr Mills, was initially enthusiastic about referring him. He now seems to have gone cold on this. Nonetheless, **JS has been awarded Legal Aid, who will pay for the investigations**[86] and this is in hand..."*

In the event, this funding source was not necessary since his investigations were paid for by the NHS. The clinical records of Child JS show that Walker-Smith knew that at least one child was in receipt of legal aid for the purpose of funding his investigation in November 1996.

I then had a meeting on January 21, 1997, with the clinical team as part of a joint Tuesday interdepartmental meeting attended by Walker-Smith and Murch, where I informed them that I had agreed to act as an expert in the MMR litigation.

This was followed up by a letter from me to Walker-Smith on February 3, 1997, reiterating my position with respect to acting as an expert and describing my reasons for agreeing to act in this capacity. This letter was read into the evidence by me at the GMC hearing with Deer in attendance. The evidence was as follows:

> **Coonan:** *...was the question of you acting as an expert in litigation ever raised with your clinical colleagues?*
>
> *A: We had a meeting in January 1997 where the issue was discussed. My clinical colleagues were, in fairness, very reluctant to become involved in*

litigation in any form. I perfectly appreciated that.

Q: Who was present at the meeting?

A: My memory is that Professor Walker-Smith and Simon Murch were there. I will be advised or corrected but I do not remember specifically who else was there. I believe others may have been there...

Q: I am going to ask you to produce an exchange of correspondence relating to this discussion... Would you be so kind as to read this out? It is your letter.

A: Certainly.

"Dear John

re: Enterocolitis and regressive autism

Further to our meeting on Tuesday 21 January, I thought it important to write to you to clarify my role in the legal issues. I fully appreciate your desire not to become involved in the legal aspect of these cases, but I feel that it is important to express the reasons that I do feel obliged to become involved.

The future for the children with whom we are dealing is very bleak indeed. Not only are the provisions for these children within the community inadequate at present, but looking ahead to the future, there will come a time when the parents of these children die, and the patients, as chronically disabled adults, left to fend for themselves in an extremely hostile world. Were there any long-term institutions left for such children, then that is where they would end up. Since these hospitals are being closed on an almost weekly basis around the country, these hopeless individuals will be left to 'care in the community'. One does not like to imagine how it will all end. Maybe their only hope is in people taking the possible organic basis of their disease seriously enough to investigate it and institute the appropriate therapies where possible.

Vaccination is designed to protect the majority, and it does so at the expense of a minority of individuals who suffer adverse consequences. Although the case against MMR is far from proven, it is one that we are obliged to investigate in view of the consistent history given by these patients' parents and by the observations made in the United States. If this disease is caused by the MMR vaccination, then these children are *the few unfortunates that have been sacrificed to protect the majority of children in this country. If this is the case, our society has an absolute obligation to compensate and care for those who have been damaged by the vaccine for the greater good. This is an inescapable moral imperative and is the principal reason that I have decided to become involved in helping these children pursue their claims. I have considered this issue in great depth and, whilst it may not be the wish of others within the group to become involved, it falls to me to make sure that their legal cases are presented in the best possible light. Fortunately, this is entirely consistent with best clinical practice which, I believe, you are providing for these children. I felt it important, however, to let you know of my feelings on this, and the position that I feel I am obliged to adopt to support these children. Without our help, I genuinely believe that the medical profession would otherwise put them to one side, as it appears to have done in many cases already. My present fears for these children are much less than the horrible imaginings if they do not receive the appropriate help that is due to them at this stage. However, I am an optimist, and I believe that this project will turn out to be both enlightening and rewarding for all those who have been involved, and I am most grateful for your help and encouragement.*

Kindest regards & best wishes,

Yours sincerely"

Q: *Did Professor Walker-Smith reply to your letter on 20 February 1997, with a copy to Dr Murch?*

A: *Yes.*

Q: *Dr Wakefield, I think you may have dealt with this already, but so that the Panel has your response in the round in the light of your answers, was there any way in which your involvement with the Legal Aid Board was kept secret?*

A: *No.*

But again with Deer...

What has not been reported is that the nature of the project had been visualised before any of the children were even admitted to the Royal Free.

> *In June 1996 – the month before Child One's arrival at the hospital – Wakefield and Barr filed a confidential document with the government's Legal Aid Board, appearing already to know of a "new syndrome".*

The document to which Deer refers[87] describes a research proposal for detecting measles virus in biopsy tissues. It involved the analysis of biopsies from five children with Crohn's disease, where there is a well-established intestinal disease, and five children with autistic regression and intestinal symptoms. This was a completely separate piece of work from *The Lancet* paper.

The document states the following in paragraph 3, page 1:

> *Briefly these conditions consist of Crohn's disease (and inflammatory bowel disease); there are also persistent reports of children suffering symptoms akin to autism (here described as disintegrative disorder) coupled with inflammatory bowel disease.*

The document only makes reference to reports of symptoms and makes no claim to the existence of the syndrome that was described in *The Lancet* paper, i.e., "ileocolonic lymphoid nodular hyperplasia, nonspecific colitis and pervasive developmental disorder in children."

The document makes it clear in paragraph 3, page 2, that what distinguishes the children with Crohn's disease and those with the putative enteritis/ disintegrative disorder syndrome is the presence of "a prima facie gastrointestinal pathology" in the children with Crohn's disease. Deer's claim seeks to convey the impression that I was "aware" of the syndrome eventually described in *The Lancet* paper before children with the *possible* syndrome were ever investigated and, hence, I had predetermined that it would be present.

> *Referring to inflammatory bowel disease, and then bowel problems with autism, Wakefield and Barr wrote to the board, successfully seeking money.*
>
> *"The objective," they wrote, "is to seek evidence which will be acceptable in a court of law of the causative connection between either the mumps, measles and rubella vaccine or the measles/rubella vaccine and certain conditions which have been reported with considerable frequency by families who are seeking compensation."*

It was made clear during the GMC hearing[88] that Barr was responsible for describing the legal aspects of this submission to the Legal Aid Board and, accordingly, it was he who wrote the paragraph above.

Twenty months later, the Royal Free team delivered the paper that had found a "new syndrome".

The "new syndrome" that Deer refers to could only have been described *after* the children had been investigated and could not have been anticipated in June 1996. At that stage (June 1996) the evidence for a possible syndrome was the *symptoms*, i.e., autistic regression and inflammatory bowel disease. The syndrome that was ultimately described is the combination of autistic regression and intestinal inflammation. Deer conflates the former with latter. In doing so, he leads the reader into believing that I had already made up my mind about the final syndrome as early as June 1996, before the children had ever been investigated.

Today, the 12 children are mostly teenagers. At least three are bloggers, two in support of Wakefield, while others have limited skills. The wrongful stigma of disability hangs heavy on most, and heaviest on the families with the misguided burden of guilt that the vaccine scare has visited on them.

Wakefield has left Britain to live in Austin, Texas, where he runs a clinic offering colonoscopies to American children. He tours the country, giving lectures and speeches against the vaccine, and attracting a loyal following of young mothers.

In Wakefield's view, the Lancet paper was accurate, including reasonable reassessment of findings. Other doctors, including an experienced pathologist concurred with his judgment on the revised reports of nonspecific colitis, he has said.

False: In fact it is I who have concurred with the judgment of others – qualified histopathologists who generated the revised reports – not the other way around as Deer's article reports.

Behavioural diagnoses, meanwhile, involved a confusing array of technical names, and he trusted what the parents told him. The fact that they said the problems followed MMR implied that regression was involved.

False: I was not responsible for making a clinical diagnosis of the behavioral disorder, on the one hand, nor on the other, determining, whether regression had occurred and, if so, whether MMR was the trigger. *The Lancet* paper documents the basis for making the developmental diagnoses: this required a full clinical history, reference to records of early development, and in the majority of children, review by a child psychiatrist.

> *Many of the parents of the original 12 children continue to support him and campaign vigorously on his behalf. But others whose children took part in the Lancet project are too burdened and traumatised for campaigning.*

At least in this, Deer is correct.

The Source

What gave Deer the unqualified gall, the verbal swagger, to challenge experts in the field of pathology and pediatric bowel disease in the popular press? Part of the answer, at least, is *another* expert in bowel disease – Professor Tom MacDonald from St. Bartholemew's. MacDonald is not a clinician, not a pathologist, but a scientist. Working previously as part of Walker-Smith's team, he did not make the journey to the Royal Free when his professor's team transferred in 1995. In the MMR litigation, both in the US and the UK, he acted as an expert for the defendants.

The GMC vetted MacDonald as a potential witness against me and his erstwhile colleagues. The attendance note of his meeting with GMC lawyers in 2005 reads:

> He [MacDonald] *believes Wakefield is a charlatan, who has been pursuing his own agenda since 1995, this being to win the Nobel Prize. He believes Wakefield's alleged link between measles vaccine and Crohn's was entirely fabricated in order to obtain publicity for this reason.*[92]

With respect to the autism question, it is my sincere belief that, as a source for Deer, MacDonald's contempt for me and for the notion of bowel disease in children with autism is captured in the following memo to Deer. The memo itself refers to a colonoscopy video, presumably from one of *The Lancet 12*:

> *Of course, when this* [video] *was made, Wakefield already thought he had the Nobel prize in his grasp because he thought he saw measles virus in the big lymphoid follicles in the ileum… However when you see the video, you can see that it is virtually impossible to biopsy the*

ileum without biopsying a lymphoid follicle. If you then decide that on histology tissue section [down the microscope], the presence of a follicle is pathology, then you end up with how Wakefield can claim that 88.5%[89] of the children had ileal pathology. **It is a deliberate deception.**[90]

Other than a preoccupation with the Nobel Prize, MacDonald – if it is he – fails to explain to Deer why biopsies from the ileum of non-autistic children (in which it would be equally "virtually impossible" to miss a lymphoid follicle) did not show the same changes as the children with autism. He may also have failed to disclose conflicting agendas, one scientific (as above) and one personal; as related to me by John Walker-Smith, when MacDonald declined the invitation to transfer to the Royal Free with Walker-Smith, he had reportedly vowed to his boss to destroy my career.[91] Deer has been useful to him in that respect.

Postscript
A complaint has been made to the UK's Press Complaints Commission (PCC) about Deer's reportage. In their response to this complaint, lawyers acting for *The Sunday Times* considered that a full response to the details of the complaint would be too onerous at this stage. Despite the fact that the matters covered in the complaint did not form part of the GMC's case (and findings) against me, the PCC deferred action on the complaint until after the GMC process was complete. The PCC did require that Deer's articles be removed from *The Sunday Times* website. In defiance of the PCC, the articles were reinstated when a press release was issued that highlighted the PCC's directive. The PCC's failure to enforce their directive is not reassuring.

Endnotes

¹ E-mail from Alistair Brett, in-house lawyer for *The Sunday Times*, to Abel Hadden of Bell-Pottinger. June 18, 2004.

² Wakefield AJ, Murch SH, Anthony A, Linnell J, Casson DM, Malik M, Berelowitz M, Dhillon AP, Thomson MA, Harvey P, Valentine A, Davies SE, Walker-Smith JA. Ileal lymphoid nodular hyperplasia, non-specific colitis and pervasive developmental disorder in children. *The Lancet.* 1998;351:637-641. [retracted]

³ Deer's allegation to the GMC regarding unethical experimentation: Letter of Deer to Tim Cox-Brown February 25, 2004, p. 3. "Therefore, there was, in my view, neither ethical approval, nor clinical indication for the invasive investigation of some children."

⁴ Walker-Smith JA. Statement. *The Lancet.* 2004;363:822-823.

⁵ See statement of Dr. Dhillon below, footnote 16.

⁶ Wakefield AJ. Autistic enterocolitis: is it a histological entity? *Histopathology.* 2006;50:380-384.

⁷ Wakefield AJ, Murch SH, Anthony A, Linnell J, Casson DM, Malik M, Berelowitz M, Dhillon AP, Thomson MA, Harvey P, Valentine A, Davies SE, Walker-Smith JA. Ileal lymphoid nodular hyperplasia, non-specific colitis and pervasive developmental disorder in children. *The Lancet.* 1998;351:637-641. [retracted]

⁸ Dr. Sue Davies, consultant histopathologist, Royal Free Hospital.

⁹ Amar P. Dhillon, Andrew Anthony, Andrew Wakefield.

¹⁰ Wakefield AJ, Anthony A, Murch SH. Enterocolitis in children with developmental disorders. *American Journal of Gastroenterology.* 2000; 95;2285–2295.

Enterocolitis in Children With Developmental Disorders

> *Mucosal biopsies were taken from the ileum, cecum/ascending colon, transverse colon, descending/sigmoid colon, and rectum. Hematoxylin and eosin-stained histological sections from all biopsies were reviewed in the routine pathology laboratory, followed by independent review and scoring on a standard proforma (Table 1)[10]. In those cases where there was disagreement between these two reports, sections were examined and reported by a third senior pathologist, whose arbitration provided the final score. In an identical manner, histological sections from the ileum and colon of children without developmental disorder were scored (median age 11.5 years; range 2-13). These included 22 consecutive ileocolonoscopic biopsy series that had been reported as normal after routine histopathology assessment. All children in this non-IBD control group had undergone ileocolonoscopy for investigation of intestinal symptoms and are included in the 37 endoscopic controls, as described above. To validate further the evaluation and scoring, 10 coded ileocolonic biopsy series (five affected children and five non-IBD controls) were reviewed at another institution by a senior pathologist in an observer-blinded fashion. Data from these independent assessments were compared.*

¹¹ *Results. Ten ileocolonic biopsy series were reviewed and scored in an observer-blinded fashion at an independent institution. No indication was given of how many samples came from each patient group. Cases [autistic children's biopsies] were clearly distinguished from controls [non-autistic children's biopsies] by the blinded reviewer[11]. Out of a possible total of 15 points, independent scores were identical for the same criterion in four of 10 cases (40%), within one point of each other in five of 10 cases (50%), and within two points of each other in one of 10 cases (10%) (Spearman rank correlation 0.79; p < 0.006). No reviewer scored systematically higher or lower than the other.*

¹² Wakefield AJ. Autistic enterocolitis: is it a histological entity? *Histopathology.* 2006;50:380-384. This was an invited response to a paper by MacDonald and Domizio that questioned the validity of the bowel disorder in autistic children. [*Histopathology*; same volume as above.]

Autistic enterocolitis: is it a histopathological entity?

For the purpose of clarification, children with developmental disorder were seen in the Department of Paediatric Gastroenterology at the Royal Free for evaluation of their gastrointestinal symptoms. Definitive and appropriate assessment included ileo-colonoscopy, upper gastrointestinal endoscopy and histopathology. Biopsy specimens were subjected to routine assessment by the duty pathologist and subsequent detailed review with scoring on a semiquantitative scale as illustrated in the manuscript of MacDonald and Domizio. The proforma was designed by Professor A. Dhillon of the Department of Histopathology, who with Dr A. Anthony evaluated the sections for the purposes of completion of this proforma. The interobserver variation using the histopathology proforma was high and is described in detail.1 Both pathologists have an extensive, published track record in mucosal histopathology. In addition, all diagnoses were routinely reviewed at a weekly clinicopathological meeting involving clinicians and pathologists, and frequently modified as a consequence.

[13] GMC vs Wakefield, Walker-Smith, and Murch. Dr. Wakefield's evidence. Tr. 49

Coonan: *I want to come on now to what you, in anticipation, describe as "Research tests", and we see that under the heading of "intestinal biopsy research" there are references in the right-hand column on page 221 to histology, and we see that on the first page of this document, in the fourth column down, there was also a reference to histology. Why is histology captured under this heading of "Research tests" with the source reference at page 221? What is the difference between the two?*

Wakefield: *Standard routine histopathology is involved in the clinical diagnosis of disease in these children. Dr Paul Dhillon as part of his contribution to this decided at a relatively early stage that, in light of the findings in these children, in light of the apparent novelty and subtlety of some of the changes, a pro forma driven analysis would be necessary in order to provide a semi quantitative estimate of what was going on in their intestine, and to this end he designed a histology pro forma which could be scored as, for example, zero for no inflammation; one for mild inflammation; two for moderate inflammation, and three for severe inflammation, and he took the various categories of changes in the intestine and set them out under those numbers, normal, mild, moderate and severe. And that was used in a detailed histopathological review by Dr Dhillon and Dr Anthony, principally, with me looking over their shoulders to learn, and that formed the basis of the research histopathology.*

Coonan: *So we have, is this right, Dr Wakefield, a strata of clinical histopathology but also a strata of research histopathology?*

Wakefield: *Correct.*

And on Day 50:

Coonan: *I have two other short matters to deal with. When it came to the drafting of The Lancet paper, can we just identify together the materials that you would have had available? First of all, would you have had the referral letters?*

Wakefield: *Yes.*

Coonan: *Would you have had the clinical notes generated at the Royal Free, including correspondence to and from the Royal Free?*

Wakefield: *Yes.*

Coonan: *Would you have had the clinical histopathology documentation generated by the histopathologist including Dr Davis?*

Wakefield: *Yes...*

Coonan: *Would you have had the product of any Friday afternoon amendments in the notes?*

Wakefield: *Yes.*

Coonan: *We have heard about the role of Dr Dhillon. Did you have the product of Dr*

Dhillon in relation to this child prior to the drafting of The Lancet paper?

Wakefield: Yes, indeed; Dr Dhillon's detailed research, overview, in the pro forma driven format that I have talked about last week was available and in fact was the final determinant of the diagnosis in these children.

Coonan: Just for completeness, would you take volume 7 of the Panel bundles, and look at tab 16? In general terms, what is tab 16?

Wakefield: Some time during the course of the investigation of these children it became clear that there was a possible new syndrome emerging, that bowel disease was indeed being found, immunological abnormalities were being found. By way of our training in academic medicine, which is largely pro forma driven and database driven, it was felt appropriate to develop a system, albeit rather primitive at the time, to make sure that all the relevant information was being captured. This is not necessarily a research exercise, although it can be; it is a way of making sure that you have ticked the boxes, that you have captured the relevant information in a consistent way across a group of patients. So this is a pro forma or these are draft pro formas in various states of preparation the design of which was mine. What I have attempted to do in this is to capture the salient features of his child's history, the demographic information, their infancy, their childhood development, their infectious and vaccine exposure, their histology and so on and so forth.

Coonan: Did it include the product from Dr Dhillon?

Wakefield: Yes. If you turn to page 243, you will see an example of the histology pro forma that I mentioned to you. Now this is a summary pro forma. Each individual biopsy, and there may be seven or eight of them from the colon of a particular child, has one page like this. You will see the designation down the left hand column of: acute inflammation, chronic inflammation, epithelial or laminar propria changes, et cetera. These are just histological matters of interest. Then across the top, if there were none of these features of interest present, there was a zero score. If they were present and mild, then a score of 1, moderate 2, severe 3, and then a total score given. This is Dr Dhillon's contribution to this work. This was done in co operation with Dr Andrew Anthony.

[14] Signed statement of Dr. A.P. Dhillon to the GMC.

17. In quite a different way [to routine diagnostic histopathology], when a histopathologist provides systematic observations for research purposes, it is best practice to be unbiased and not to see the clinical details of the patient who has provided the sample. In the context of inflammatory bowel disease, the histopathologist might put more order into his observations and may say whether there is acute inflammation, chronic inflammation, ulceration, or architectural changes. He/she will also comment on the extent to which these things can be seen on the slide. Histopathologists sometimes record their observations as a "score" ranging 0-III, where '0' could represent no inflammation, 'I' could represent mild inflammation, 'II' could represent moderate inflammation, and 'III' could represent severe inflammation.

18. I often use this type of scoring system when I am asked to undertake a systematic review for research purposes. I will look at each slide down the microscope and record the relevant features for each slide in a table. I may record a score for some of the relevant microscopical features in the table as well.

19. The different scores of 0-III representing for example, different degrees of inflammation, are not necessarily reproduced in a published research paper unless a specific referee requests it.

20. My appointment in the Medical School requires me to undertake research activities. Around 1997, I was asked by Dr Wakefield to review a series of slides of gut biopsies from patients from the paediatric gastroenterology department. …Biopsies would have been taken from different parts of the gut from each patient, and I would have looked at the whole series of biopsies for each patient.

21. For my research review of slides, I was not given any clinical details about the

children who had provided the samples. I made microscopical observations and recorded these observations using the system described above. The observations were given to Dr Wakefield.

22. When I was asked to do this review of slides, I did not know what symptoms the children had. The review of the slides was straightforward and was a matter of saying whether there was inflammation or not as well as other relevant microscopical observations.

23. The idea to publish the series of children described in the 1998 Lancet paper had arisen probably in 1997. It was then that I learned more about the clinical syndrome which the children (included in the slide series which I had reviewed) apparently had. My clinical colleagues told me that this was a group of children with a syndrome that included gut problems, endoscopic changes and a particular histological appearance. These children had delayed or regressed development. The syndrome became more coherent to me when I saw a draft of the paper.

24. The paper contained histology paragraphs and a table which includes a column where the histological findings for the 12 children have been written up. I did not write the histology section of the paper and I cannot remember whether I made any amendments to the draft paper which would have been circulated to all of the authors. I do not know if any other histopathologists undertook the same review exercise with the slides as me, and I did not see their observations.

25. The person who wrote the histological findings may have looked at the observations which I provided to Dr Wakefield. The person writing the research paper may have translated the Roman numeral scores which I may have used into something readable. For example, the term "lymphoid nodular hyperplasia" is synonymous with "increased or enlarged lymphoid follicles", and this in aspect of chronic inflammation.

26. The paper was published in the Lancet in February 1998 and was entitled "Ileal-lymphoid nodular hyperplasia, non-specific colitis, and pervasive developmental disorder in children" ("the Lancet paper"). I was named as one of the authors on this paper because of the blinded review of the series of slides which I undertook in a research capacity.

[15] Gonzalez L, et al. Endoscopic and Histological Characteristics of the Digestive Mucosa in Autistic Children with gastro-Intestinal Symptoms. *Arch Venez Pueric Pediatr*, 2005;69:19-25.

Balzola F, et al. Panenteric IBD-like disease in a patient with regressive autism shown for the first time by wireless capsule enteroscopy: Another piece in the jig-saw of the gut-brain syndrome? *American Journal of Gastroenterology*, 2005. 100(4):979- 981.

Krigsman A, et al. http://www.cevs.ucdavis.edu/Cofred/Public/Aca/WebSec.cfm?confid=238&webid=1245 (last accessed June 2007) [no longer available; full paper now published below as footnote 16]. Balzola F, et al. Autistic enterocolitis: confirmation of a new inflammatory bowel disease in an Italian cohort of patients. *Gastroenterology* 2005;128(Suppl. 2);A-303.

[16] Galiatsatos P, Gologan A, Lamoureux E. Autistic enterocolitis: fact or fiction. *Canadian Journal of Gastroenterology*. 2009;23:95-98.

Krigsman A, Boris M, Goldblatt A, Stott C. Clinical Presentation and Histologic Findings at Ileocolonoscopy in Children with Autistic Spectrum Disorder and Chronic Gastrointestinal Symptoms. *Autism Insights*. 2009;1:1–11.

Chen B, Girgis S, El-Matary W. Childhood autism and eosinophilic colitis. *Digestion*. 2010;81:127-9. Epub 2010 Jan 9.

[17] Taylor B, Miller E, Farrington CP, Petropoulos MC, Favot-Mayaud I, Li J, Waight PA. Autism and measles, mumps, and rubella vaccine: No epidemiological evidence for a causal association. *The Lancet*. 1999;353:2026-9.

[18] Wakefield AJ. MMR vaccination and autism. *The Lancet*, 1999;354:949-950.

[19] Clinic note of Professor Walker-Smith, June 20, 1996. Royal Free Hospital records.

[20] Wakefield AJ, Murch SH, Anthony A, Linnell J, Casson DM, Malik M, Berelowitz M, Dhillon AP, Thomson MA, Harvey P, Valentine A, Davies SE, Walker-Smith JA. Ileal lymphoid nodular hyperplasia, non-specific colitis and pervasive developmental disorder in children. *The Lancet* 1998;351:637-641. [retracted]

[21] General practice records, p. 54.

[22] General practice records, p. 6.

[23] "Hearing" followed by a horizontal arrow which designates "normal" in medical clerking.

[24] General practice records, p.14.

[25] [Age 2 months] Health visitor record.

[26] [Age 7 months] Health visitor record.

[27] Dr. Mark Berelowitz letter to Dr. Simon Murch. September 30, 1996. Royal Free Hospital records, pp. 143-144.

[28] Emphasis added.

[29] Royal Free Hospital records, p. 145.

[30] Royal Free Hospital records, p. 25.

[31] Royal Free Hospital records, p. 143.

[32] Letter from Dr. Robert Surtees, pediatric neurologist at Great Ormond Street Hospital, to Dr. Hilary Cass at Harper House. August 23, 1996. General practitioner records, p. 146.

[33] East Suffolk Health Authority discharge note. March 16, 1993: "febrile convulsion"

[34] Health Visitor Records. p. 3.

[35] Letter from Dr. Casson to Dr. Bennett, community pediatrician. May 19, 1997. Royal Free Hospital Records, p. 80.

[36] Lack of eye contact is a cardinal feature of autism.

[37] Health visitor records, December 21, 1994.

[38] General practice records p. 23.

[39] General practice records p. 24. "Development N" (circled) standing for "normal."

[40] General practice records p. 296.

[41] General practice records p. 296.

[42] Local hospital records pp. 111-112.

[43] General practice records, p. 28 – "autism". File RFH17 – diagnosed with autism at age 3 years by Bennett (community pediatrician).

[44] Correspondence from JWS to Dr. Nalletamby summarizing Child 6 as within the autistic spectrum and having chronic bowel symptoms. February10, 1996.

[45] General practice records, p. 244 – reference to regressive nature of the problem. General practice records, p. 309 – sequence of regression described in detail.

[46] General practice records, p. 218 – no concern about early developmental milestones.

[47] General practice records p. 86 – at 21 months saying 3-4 word sentences, following MMR speech stopped – "flat effect," "completely babyish."

General practice records p. 219 – regression in language skills at about 2.5 years (see also GPR220).

General practice records p. 357 – Professor Neville: behaviour a problem at 20 months, after MMR. "Stopped speaking and lost bowel control."

General practice records p. 279 – letter from Professor Walker-Smith: mother gives history of fit following MMR and changes in behavior.

[48] General practice records p. 222 – September 1998: diagnosed with "Pathological Demand Avoidance in the autistic spectrum" (see also GPR230).

General practice records p. 276 – February 1997 –GP thinks he has "autism/autistic spectrum."

General practice records p. 239 – "diagnosis of autistic spectrum disorder somewhere between high functioning autism and Asperger's."

General practice records p. 59 – "autistic spectrum" diagnosis.

General practice records p. 417 – "pervasive developmental disorder."

General practice records p. 353 – "pervasive developmental disorder."

General practice records p. 222 – "pervasive developmental disorder in the autistic spectrum."

General practice records pp. 135, 141, 163, 169, 189, 239, 276, 357. General consensus by early 1997 that Child 7 has autism spectrum disorder.

[49] Confirmed in letter from Dr. Houlsby to Dr. Tapsfield, attached to statement of Dr. Jelly.

[50] Royal Free Hospital discharge summary, January 27, 1997, attached to statement of Dr. Jelly.

[51] General practice records, p. 25.

[52] Confirmed in letter from Dr. Houlsby to Dr. Tapsfield, attached to statement of Dr. Jelly and letter to Dr. Hunter from Dr. Houlsby, December 23, 1994: "felt that her abilities although delayed on the average age of attainment were not outside the range of normal."

[53] Royal Free Hospital records, p. 7. January 19, 1996.

[54] Royal Free Hospital records, p. 21.

[55] Dr. Jelly statement to GMC, Day 29.

[56] General practice records, p. 94.

[57] General practice records p. 25 – "MMR Jan 95, grand mal convulsion Feb 95 2 weeks after MMR, never the same again."

General practice records, p. 76 – discharge letter from RFH: "dramatic deterioration" from 18 months.

General practice records, p. 83 – GP letter: some developmental delay before MMR but "mother adamant that she lost her speech after MMR."

General practice records, p. 94 – at 17 months she was within the lower range of normal, at 20 months she was globally developmentally delayed functioning at about a "one year level."

General practice records, p. 111 – letter from GP: "regression after MMR."

General practice records, p. 120 – loss of speech shown on video.

General practice records, p. 121 – clear evidence of regression prior to admission.

General practice records, p. 127 – concern over lack of speech (although continued to say a few words).

General practice records, p. 130 – mother associates "setback" with MMR.

General practice records, p. 131 – letter from pediatrician: "at one year level on Denver Developmental Assessment."

General practice records, p. 133 – letter from pediatric cardiologist: no speech whereas previously said single words.

General practice records, p. 136 – evidence of regression.

General practice records, p. 139 –evidence of regression.

General practice records, p. 142 – her speech has regressed.

Royal Free Hospital records, p. 7 – admitted with history of developmental delay following dramatic deterioration.

Royal Free Hospital records, p. 17 – letter to AW from Dr. Berney: appears to accept abrupt post MMR regression.

Royal Free Hospital records, p. 18 – mother reports "catastrophic deterioration" post MMR. "Became a different person."

Royal Free Hospital records, p. 20 – history of dramatic deterioration in referral to Berelowitz.

Royal Free Hospital records, p. 49 – good evidence of regression.

Local hospital records, p. 20 – accepts that there were concerns re development prior to MMR but then makes clear that there was a subsequent deterioration.

Local hospital records, p. 45 – further evidence of regression.

[58] GMC vs Wakefield, Walker-Smith, and Murch. Evidence of Dr Jelley. Tr. 29.

[59] GMC vs Wakefield, Walker-Smith, and Murch. Tr. 29:

> [Child 8's] *mother came to the Genetics clinic recently without* [Child 8]. *Unfortunately we are still unable to reach a firm diagnosis to explain* [Child 8's] *developmental delay, coarctation of the aorta and slightly unusual face. Her mother reports that she is still without speech.*
>
> *Much of our discussion recently centered around* [Child 8's] *mother's concerns that her problems stemmed from her MMR vaccination at 19 months. She tells me that a couple of weeks after the injection she developed a measles rash and was very poorly with it. She subsequently fitted and was admitted to hospital where she was found to be dehydrated.* [Child's 8] *mother is aware that there may be an underlying cause for* [Child 8's] *problems but is obviously also anxious that the MMR injection either caused her developmental delay or exacerbated it. She has been in touch with an organisation Jabs [sic] and is in contact with a mother of a child who similarly feels that her child's problems date from the MMR immunisation. Interestingly* [Child 8's] *mother feels very strongly that* [Child 8's] *speech was coming on well before she had her immunisation and that she had several words at that stage which she subsequently lost.*

[60] Histopathology is the process of making a microscopic diagnosis on tissues taken from a patient.

[61] Royal Free Hospital records, p. 61.

[62] Royal Free Hospital records, p. 15.

[63] Proforma report of Child 8.

[64] Royal Free Hospital records, p. 48.

[65] In his evidence to the GMC on Day 81, page 12, Walker-Smith was questioned:

> **Stephen Miller QC:** *We have got up to 11 December 1996. You have told the Panel in general terms and in relation to individual children about the review of histology which you carried out with Dr Dhillon?*
>
> **Walker-Smith:** *Yes.*
>
> **Miller:** *In December 1996, so in the period with which we are now concerned, in which we are looking at this child's investigation. Was this child one of the children whose histology you reviewed with Dr Dhillon after he did his blinded assessment of the slides?*
>
> **Walker-Smith:** *Yes.*
>
> **Miller:** *If we look at the penultimate page in the clip that we have, D14. Professor, just under half way down in that note of the way you deal with a brief summary of the history, then the blood results. Then, under "Endoscopy," what have you written?*
>
> **Walker-Smith:** *I have written:*
>
> *"Lymphoid nodular hyperplasia terminal ileum."*
>
> **Miller:** *Then "Histology" underneath that?*
>
> **Walker-Smith:** *I have written:*

"Prominent lymphoid follicles

Dhillon – moderate to mild increase in intra epithelial lymphocytes. Increase in chronic inflammatory cells through the colon – superficial macrophages not quite granuloma".

Then my overall clinical opinion:

"Indeterminate colitis."

[66] GMC vs Wakefield, Walker-Smith and Murch Tr. 81, p. 13.

Miller: *"Histologically there was an increase in chronic inflammatory cells throughout the colon with a moderate increase in intra-epithelial lymphocytes."*

Walker-Smith: *Yes.*

Miller: *Again, putting that alongside what you have said in this handwritten note at D14, is that taken from that handwritten note?*

Walker-Smith: *It is.*

Miller: *Because you have said:*

"Moderate to marked increase in intra-epithelial lymphocytes. Increase in chronic inflammatory cells throughout the colon."

[67] Child 9 draft proforma report.

[68] Royal Free Hospital records, Vol. 2, p. 47.

[69] GMC vs Wakefield, Walker-Smith and Murch. Tr. 81.

Miller: *If we look at 59A it sets out what the original finding was of Dr Jarmulowicz. Then microscopic description supplementary report at the bottom of the page.*

Walker-Smith: *Yes.*

Miller: *These biopsies have been reviewed following a clinicopathological meeting. The ileal biopsy shows confluent lymphoid aggregates within otherwise unremarkable small intestine. The large bowel biopsies show a very subtle scattering of chronic inflammatory cells within the lamina propria. The superficial lamina propria contains focal nuclear debris and the surface epithelium appears slightly degenerate. No active inflammation is seen. More levels have been cut and no granulomas have been identified.*

Comment: Minor abnormalities. ? Significance."

And that is countersigned on this occasion by Dr Davies as well as by Dr Jarmulowicz.

Walker-Smith: *Yes.*

Miller: *What, if anything, is the difference between those two sets of findings?*

Walker-Smith: *The principal difference really is in the large bowel report – a very subtle scattering of chronic inflammatory cells within the lamina propria is a clear indication of chronic inflammation. And the so-called focal nuclear debris, that tells us that there has been some damage in the past; and the surface epithelium said to be slightly degenerate also tells us that there has been some damage, but there is no evidence of active inflammation. Curiously, this report actually leaves out an important observation which Dr Jarmulowicz made in the first report, saying that the lymphoid tissue shows reactive changes, which I regard as rather important.*

Miller: *The conclusion from the second report, the amended or updated report is:*

"Minor abnormalities? Significance."

Who makes the decision as to the interpretation overall of the abnormalities, if there are abnormalities, on the slides?

Walker-Smith: *The clinician.*

Miller: *How does that work? You have a report from a histopathologist in which he sets out in detail what the findings are for individual sections, or groups of sections, and then comes to his conclusion; but in terms of the management of the patient how does the decision get made?*

Walker-Smith: *The histology report gives the objective evidence of things that are seen down the microscope in a descriptive term. The histopathologists do offer their opinion as to possible significance, but the clinician is the person responsible for putting together the clinical features – that is the signs and the symptoms – the endoscopic features and the observed histopathological features.*

Miller: *If we look at Dr Casson's note at page 17 in volume 2. We have seen the top half of this note before, which is written on the printed form for endoscopy – it is under histology.*

"Colonic biopsies – normal crypt architecture; very mild distribution of chronic inflammatory cells. Decreased goblet cells. Focal abnormalities of epithelium, i.e. tufting. Nuclear debris in sub-epithelium deposits."

Walker-Smith: *Yes.*

Miller: *That is again a slightly different description.*

Walker-Smith: *Yes.*

Miller: *But in what circumstances would that have been written?*

Walker-Smith: *Presumably that was written by David Casson at the time of the histopathological meeting as a record as he saw it.*

Miller: *Then at the last line he does those arrows leading from one thing to another, so there is an arrow and then:*

"Enough chronic inflammation to merit treatment with sulphasalazine."

Walker-Smith: *I think this might be a quotation from myself.*

Miller: *Perhaps you could explain how it comes about?*

Walker-Smith: *Usually I and my two consultant colleagues would come to a view as to the clinical significance of the findings which we observed at the clinicopathological meeting because one of the junior doctors did in fact present the history and findings. Then the relevant consultant endoscopist would tell us about the endoscopic findings; then we would see in front of us on the screen what the histopathology was. Then the clinicians and indeed the junior doctors would discuss together what was the way forward because the parents are usually waiting in the ward after the meeting, and Dr Casson would go and speak to them. I believed on the total picture that it was appropriate to use sulphasalazine and, although it is not written there, I was obviously making a diagnosis of indeterminate colitis.*

[70] Proforma report of Child 10.
[71] Emphasis added.
[72] Royal Free Hospital records, pp. 86 and 87.
[73] JWS presentation to Wellcome Trust meeting, December 1996.
[74] Proforma report of Child 3.
[75] Royal Free Hospital records, p. 27.
[76] General practice records, p. 99.
[77] Royal Free Hospital records, p. 35.
[78] Royal Free Hospital records, pp. 35 and 36.
[79] GMC vs Wakefield, Walker-Smith, and Murch. Tr. 53.

Coonan: *Thank you very much. Can I turn from medical matters and research matters to the question of legal aid? There is a reference to legal aid that I would like you to look at in volume 1 of the Panel bundle at page 242. This is a legal aid certificate for Child 12 and for my purposes the only thing I need from this is the date, at the bottom right-hand corner, 9 October 1996. Did you ever get to know that this child had a legal aid certificate?*

Wakefield: *Yes.*

Q: *When did you get to know that?*

A: No, I cannot remember, but as it turns out this is the only child who was, to our knowledge involved in litigation – subsequent knowledge. It turns out that this is the only child who had a legal aid certificate prior to [errata: after] their referral and investigation at the Royal Free Hospital.

Q: But at the time of the referral or about the time of the referral and investigation did you know then that he had a legal aid certificate?

A: I have no memory of it.

Q: Did this child become one of the Legal Aid Board children?

A: Yes, I think he did.

Q: Did you have any understanding or appreciation of any litigation motivation by the mother at or about the time of referral.

A: No, the mother's motivation is evident in the letters that she has written to Professor Walker-Smith and that is the gastrointestinal symptoms and problems that she felt were present in her child.

[80] Letter from 8 of the 12 parents. December 22, 2008. One lives in the US and 2 could not be contacted. The third remaining parent sent an e-mail of support but wished to remain anonymous.

An Open Letter: To Whom It May Concern

We are writing to you as parents of the children who, because of their symptoms of inflammatory bowel disease and associated autism, were seen at the Royal Free Hospital Paediatric Gastroenterology Unit by Professor Walker-Smith and Dr Simon Murch with the involvement of Dr Andrew Wakefield on the research side of their investigations. Our children became the subjects of a paper published in The Lancet in 1998.

We know these three doctors are being investigated by the General Medical Council (GMC) on the basis of allegations made to them by a freelance reporter. Among the many allegations made are the suggestions that the doctors acted inappropriately regarding our children, that Dr Wakefield "solicited them for research purposes" and that our children had not been referred in the usual way by their own GPs. It is also claimed that our children were given unnecessary and invasive investigations for the purpose of research, and not in their interest. We know this was not so. All of our children were referred to Professor Walker-Smith in the proper way in order that their severe, long-standing and distressing gastroenterological symptoms could be fully investigated and treated by the foremost paediatric gastroenterologists in the UK. Many of us had been to several other doctors in our quest to get help for our children but not until we saw Professor Walker-Smith and his colleagues were full investigations undertaken. We were all treated with utmost professionalism and respect by all three of these doctors. Throughout our children's care at the Royal Free Hospital we were kept fully informed about the investigations recommended and the treatment plans which evolved. All of the investigations were carried out without distress to our children, many of whom made great improvements on treatment so that for the first time in years they were finally pain-free.

We have been following the GMC hearings with distress as we, the parents, have had no opportunity to refute the allegations. For the most part we have been excluded from giving evidence to support these doctors whom we all hold in very high regard. It is for this reason we are writing to the GMC and to all concerned to be absolutely clear that the complaint that is being brought against these three caring and compassionate physicians does not in any way reflect our perception of the treatment offered to our sick children at the Royal Free. We are appalled that these doctors have been the subject of this protracted enquiry in the absence of any complaint from any parent about any of the children who were reported in the Lancet paper.

[81] GMC vs Wakefield, Walker-Smith and Murch. Tr. 73.

Q: As far as you were concerned and your colleagues, Dr Murch, Dr Thomson and the junior doctors involved in your department, what was your role going to be?
A: Our role was a purely clinical role, inasmuch as we would see the children and it would be me in this particular case, I would see all of the children where possible myself in the out-patient clinic. I would then make a decision as to whether I thought the children had any kind of bowel inflammation, whether Crohn's disease or other bowel inflammation. If I thought clinically that the child required investigation on clinical grounds, I would then recommend ileocolonoscopy. Then I would also move towards considering other investigations which may be undertaken. We had formed the impression that neurological disease, which presented in a manner similar to autism, had to be excluded in these children. There had been quite a lot of discussion about this, particularly involving Dr Mike Thomson, who in our discussions had discussed this with us. These investigations were obviously clinically drawn, but we had not actually finalised precisely what was going to be the way forward at that time.

[82] Emphasis added.

[83] Jabs is the acronym for Justice and Awareness Basic Support. www.jabs.org.uk.

[84] Langdon-Down G. (1996, November 27). "Law: A shot in the Dark." *The Independent.* Page 25.

[85] Child JS, Royal Free Hospital records, p. 76.

[86] Emphasis added.

[87] Proposed Protocol and Costing Proposals for testing a selected number of MR and MMR vaccinated children. 'LAB protocol".

[88] GMC vs Wakefield, Walker-Smith and Murch. Tr. 73.

> **Coonan:** *Is that a correct way of approaching matters? That using that protocol it will be possible to establish the causal link between the administration of the vaccine and the conditions outlined in this proposed protocol and costing proposals?*
>
> **Wakefield:** *Yes. This is his document and these are his words, and they are crafted in a legal way. In other words, they are not necessarily what a scientist might say. For example, it would be possible to establish "the causal link". Now, it is more accurate to say that it would be possible to establish an association, for example, or a possible causal association, that would be scientifically more accurate, but the difference with this document is that one was dealing with a balance of probability argument, which is a legal argument and something with which I had no familiarity at all. I was used to dealing with scientific levels of proof and not balance of evidence arguments, so, as I say, these are his words, his interpretation, and it is framed in a way that would be understandable to, presumably, colleagues at the Legal Aid Board.*

[89] Wakefield AJ, Anthony A, Murch SH, Thomson M, Montgomery SM, Davis S, et al. Enterocolitis in children with developmental disorders. *Am. J. Gastroenterol.* 2000;95:2285-2295.

> *Histologically, reactive follicular hyperplasia was present in 46 of 52 (88.5%) ileal biopsies from affected children and in four of 14 (29%) with UC, but not in non-IBD controls (p < 0.01).*

[90] Emphasis added.

[91] Disclosed by Walker-Smith to AJW; personal communication.

[92] GMC vs Wakefield, Walker-Smith, and Murch. Attendance note of meeting between MacDonald and GMC lawyers. March 23, 2005.

CHAPTER THIRTEEN

Poisoning Young Minds

Like it or not, there is an unrelenting debate about whether vaccines have poisoned the minds of some children. That vaccines *may* do so is acknowledged[1] (by, among others, autism expert Professor Sir Michael Rutter[2]) and is not actually the debate at hand; the real questions are which children and how many? The base of the tsunami that is the autism epidemic – one sustained hitherto by competing arguments for the rising number of diagnoses and those invested in non-environmental causes – is no longer able to support its top.[3] In accordance with simple wave mechanics, the tsunami's slope is too great and breaking is inevitable. Breaking, for the purpose of this metaphor, extends to the shoreline's horizon, from the child to the family, to schools, to the state budget, to public confidence in health care infrastructure, and beyond.

But another form of poison has been insinuated into the collective conscious of young, able minds that threatens like an aftershock on the seabed. Although the tendrils of this poison are deeply embedded in the history of human conflict, its main roots are to be found in the propaganda of emergent Nazi Germany circa 1935. As an example, a math question to German children in schools where Jewish children were limited to 1.5 percent by 1935 and banned from education altogether by 1939, reads as follows:

> The Jews are aliens in Germany – in 1933 there were 66,060,000 inhabitants in the German Reich, of whom 499,682 were Jews. What is the percent of aliens?[4]

It was deemed important, indeed necessary, to sow the seed of anti-Semitic propaganda early into young, fertile Aryan minds. Clearly, this was just the beginning.

Recently I was provided with the text of another exam paper, this time from the UK's January 2008 national General Certificate of School Education (GCSE) biology exam (higher tier), which students were given as part of their preparation for the 2009 exams. It read as follows:

The MMR vaccine is used to protect children against measles, mumps and, rubella.

(a) *Explain, as fully as you can, how the MMR vaccine protects children from these diseases.*

(b) *Read the passage.*

Autism is a brain disorder that can result in behavioural problems. In 1998, Dr Andrew Wakefield published a report in a medical journal. Dr Wakefield and his colleagues had carried out tests on 12 autistic children. Dr Wakefield and his colleagues claimed to have found a possible link between the MMR vaccine and autism. Dr Wakefield wrote that the parents of eight of the twelve children blamed the MMR vaccine for autism. He said that symptoms of autism had started within days of vaccination. Some newspapers used parts of the report in scare stories about the MMR vaccine. As a result, many parents refused to have their children vaccinated. Dr Wakefield's research was being funded through solicitors for the twelve children. The lawyers wanted evidence to use against vaccine manufacturers.

Use information from the passage on the opposite page to answer these questions.

(i) *Was Dr Wakefield's report based on reliable scientific evidence?*

Explain the reasons for your answer.

(ii) *Might Dr Wakefield's report have been biased?*

Give the reason for your answer.

Let us pause there in order to reflect upon the question. While several quanta removed from the implications of the Reich's insidious mathematics test, the coercive subtext is the same. It was set, apparently, by teachers trained in science. It was set for children whose futures depend upon providing answers that will allow them to pass the exam, i.e., by expressing views consistent with those of the State. It is intended to embed opinion.

First, I will deconstruct the passage that the students are given to read.

Autism is a brain disorder that can result in behavioural problems.

Actually, rather than being a brain disorder, autism is a disorder that affects the brain.[5] A growing body of published evidence indicates that for many children, autism is a systemic disorder affecting the immune system, the intestine, and various metabolic processes such as those responsible for detoxification. Similarly, Pediatric Autoimmune Neuropsychiatric Disorders Associated with Streptococcal Infections (PANDAS) is a systemic disorder associated with adverse neurologic (e.g., tic disorders) and behavioral consequences (e.g., obsessive compulsive disorder) following streptococcal infections of, for example, the tonsils rather than the brains of susceptible children.

In 1998, Dr Andrew Wakefield published a report in a medical journal. Dr Wakefield and his colleagues had carried out tests on 12 autistic children.

I, and 12 other well-respected physicians and scientists, published the report that described the results of clinical tests carried out on 12 sick children who were admitted to the Royal Free Hospital under the care of a senior pediatric gastroenterologist for investigation of their clinical symptoms. An apparently novel inflammatory bowel disease was discovered and has since been confirmed in five different countries.[6] The paper was a case series (rather than an analytic study, e.g., a case-control study); this was clearly stated in the paper. It is a typical and well-established mode of presenting medical cases with similar features. It is a hypothesis-generating study that is a precursor to analytic studies in which inclusion of controls is appropriate.

Dr Wakefield and his colleagues claimed to have found a possible link between the MMR vaccine and autism.

We specifically stated in the paper that the findings did not prove an association – let alone a causal association – between MMR vaccine and the syndrome that was described.

Dr Wakefield wrote that the parents of eight of the twelve children blamed the MMR vaccine for autism.

Appropriately and accurately, we reported the parental histories of developmental regression following MMR vaccination in eight of the twelve children. No one would have suggested censoring, for example, parental reports of natural chicken pox if this is what had preceded their child's regression.

He said that symptoms of autism had started within days of vaccination.

We did not say this; we provided an account of the parental reports of the "onset of first behavioral symptoms," which had often started within days of receiving the MMR vaccine.

Some newspapers used parts of the report in scare stories about the MMR vaccine. As a result, many parents refused to have their children vaccinated.

This is misleading and without any evidential basis. Asked what vaccination strategy I would recommend, I suggested in 1998 (and now) a return to single-spaced vaccines. This recommendation was based upon extensive research by me into the safety studies of measles-containing vaccines, compiled into a report that was several hundred pages long. The conclusions of this report with respect to the inadequacy of MMR vaccine safety studies have since been endorsed by the gold-standard scientific review by the Cochrane Collaboration.[7] However, while a fall in uptake of MMR was reported following our publication, figures for the reciprocal uptake in single vaccines were not. I have contacted private UK clinics providing single vaccines, and I am informed that they have administered tens, if not hundreds, of thousands of doses, none of which are documented in the official statistics. Bizarrely, when the demand for single vaccines was at its highest, the UK government revoked the license for importation of single vaccines in August 1998, 6 months after I had made my recommendation. Parents with genuine safety concerns about MMR were denied a choice of how to protect their children: the UK government had decided to put protection of policy before protection of children. Beyond this point, vaccine uptake may genuinely have fallen, for which the government with its "our-way-or-no-way" policy must take responsibility.

Dr Wakefield's research was being funded through solicitors for the twelve children. The lawyers wanted evidence to use against vaccine manufacturers.

This is false. The allegation that *The Lancet* paper was funded by the LAB through lawyers looking to sue vaccine manufacturers was made by a freelance journalist who simply got it wrong and whose claims have now been discredited by the evidence (see Chapter 12, "Deer"). Not one single cent of LAB funding was spent on *The Lancet* report. In fact, the funding for the LAB study (a separate viral detection study) was not even available to be spent until 9 months after the children in *The Lancet* study had been investigated, their results analyzed, and the paper written and submitted to *The Lancet* for possible publication. These are matters of fact.

In other words, the students' required reading is substantially false or misleading. And yet in order to gain marks, the students, whatever their understanding of the true state of affairs, are required to endorse the errors of their examiners or fail on the question. The examiners provide a breakdown of their marking scheme:

> *Answer (i) Was Dr Wakefield's report based on reliable scientific evidence?*

> *A. No (any two from sample size small [only 12], conclusion based on hearsay from parents, only 8 parents linked autism to MMR, no control used (2 marks))*

First, the question is confusing; a report provides facts, and its conclusions (if any) are based upon evidence. The options given for a correct answer completely fail to understand the nature and purpose of a *case series* (such as Kanner's original description of autism in 11 children), which is essentially an uncontrolled report of the children's history backed up, where available in our case, by contemporaneous developmental records and GP reports, and clinical findings including a detailed analysis of the children's diseased intestinal tissues.

> *Answer (b)(ii) (yes) being paid by parents / lawyers (1 mark)*

As stated above, *The Lancet* 1998 paper was not funded in any way by lawyers. And rewarding the answer that I was being paid by "parents" is extraordinary; it not only bears no resemblance to the truth, but there is no mention of parents paying in the paragraph upon which the examiners base their question (see "Postscript" later in this chapter).

Finally, to part (a) of the exam question: "can we explain how MMR vaccine protects children from these diseases." A simple answer – one pleasing to the examiners – would be: *by the induction of specific, life-long antibody and cellular immunity that produces high herd immunity and interrupts chains of virus transmission.* While this may get a good mark, it would be false. In truth, there is much that is not known about vaccine-induced immunity. The legacy of mumps vaccination – a policy forced on reluctant public health systems in the US and UK, essentially through commercial pressures – has simply made mumps a more dangerous disease. Mumps is a trivial disease in children but substantially more dangerous in adolescents and adults. The vaccine does not protect enough children, and what protection it does confer does not last — even with boosters. The effect has been to leave pubertal and post-pubertal individuals susceptible to mumps and its complications. Measles vaccine comes considerably closer to the examiner's preferred answer, although waning immunity is also a problem that may not be overcome by booster doses, a practice that has yet to be studied adequately for safety. The long-term consequence of waning immunity at the population level is an issue of genuine concern.

I would score precisely zero for my response. But what of those who face the question in the future or who have already taken the test? The examining board was sent a series of searching questions by a journalist about this issue. Immediately, the exam paper was taken down from the website. What happens now? Will the students who have already answered the question pass if their answers conform to the dictate of the public health apparatchiks, or will they fail because their answers are wrong? And the science graduates who set the question – on what did they base their position? From their response to the journalist's questions, the answer would appear to be the integrity of *The Sunday Times* – so much for due scientific process. Where does that leave the prospects for tomorrow's medical science?

Consider the recent revelation during the course of Vioxx class action hearings: the publishing house Elsevier (owner of *The Lancet* and over 500 other medical and scientific titles) created six fake journals that were dressed up to look like scientific journals, funded by Merck without any disclosure, and strongly favorable to Merck in their content.[8] And Merck itself circulated an internal memo that suggested corporate policy on Vioxx included seeking out dissenting doctors and destroying them where they live.[9] Parents of the world's remaining neurotypical children might wish to consider this when discussing career choices.

"Corporate government" is heavily invested in propaganda, many of the techniques of which are a legacy of the Third Reich. It is difficult to believe that it was not influential in setting the UK school's biology curriculum. For their efforts, Julius Streicher,[10] the Reich's apothecary of young Aryan mind poisoning, would have given the GCSE examiners and whoever was pulling their strings no more than a six out of ten and a *"see me after class."* Streicher was tried and sentenced to death at Nuremberg. Who knows where he might otherwise have ended up?

Postscript

Sometime after this chapter originally appeared as an article in *Age of Autism*, an angry mother sent me the page of her son's AQA[11] science textbook. AQA may have been instructed that their exam-question propaganda was not damning enough, for this time they had thrown caution to the wind and had written in reference to *The Lancet* paper:

Controlling Infectious Disease

The MMR Dilemma[12]

...It turned out that the research has been done on a tiny group of twelve children. The scientist had been paid £55,000 by the parents of some of the children to prepare evidence against the vaccine for a court case. What's more, Dr Wakefield had developed some measles treatments which would not have been used if parents were confident in MMR. No one knew this when he published his results.

AQA has excelled itself: this is such utter garbage that one wonders whether Julius Streicher actually survived the hangman's noose in Nuremberg with little more than whiplash, only to return as a graying biology teacher needing to make a little money on the side. And by way of self-assessment in dystopian science, you can always go to Deer's website where you will find the following:

As taught in schools: *In 2008, Deer scored a professional first when findings from his investigation became the subject for an exam question for British **teenagers**,[13] set by the UK Assessment and Qualifications Alliance. See question 5 at this link, and, if you feel you need to, go **here** to see how you would have scored on this GCSE topic.*

Endnotes

[1] Weibel RE, et al. Acute encephalopathy followed by permanent brain injury or death associated with further attenuated measles vaccines: a review of claims submitted to the National Vaccine Injury Compensation Programme. *Pediatrics.* 1998;101:383-387.

Age of Autism. (2009, February 27) Why is the Media Ignoring the Bailey Banks Autism Vaccine Decision? Posted at http://www.ageofautism.com/2009/02/why-is-the-media-ignoring-the-bailey-banks-autism-vaccine-decision.html

[2] Rutter M, Bailey A, Bolton P, et al. Autism and known medical conditions: myth and substance. *Journal of Child Psychology and Psychiatry,* 1994; 35(2):311–22.

[3] Hertz-Picciotto, I and Delwiche, L. The rise in autism and the role of age at diagnosis. *Epidemiology,* 2009; 20:84–90; and http://www.dds.ca.gov/Autism/docs/AutismReport_2007.pdf

[4] Corelli M. (2002, May-June). Poisoning young minds in Nazi Germany: children and propaganda in the Third Reich. Retrieved from http://findarticles.com/p/articles/mi_hb6541/is_4_66/ai_n28923014/.

Herbert Hirsch, *Genocide and the Politics of Memory.* Chapel Hill: University of North Carolina Press, 1995, p. 119.

[5] Herbert M. Autism: A brain disorder, or a disorder that affects the brain? *Clinical Neuropsychiatry.* 2005;2:354-379.

[6] Wakefield AJ, Anthony A, Murch SH. Enterocolitis in children with developmental disorders. *American Journal of Gastroenterology* 2000; 95;2285–2295.

Gonzalez L, et al. Endoscopic and Histological Characteristics of the Digestive Mucosa in Autistic Children with Gastro-Intestinal Symptoms. *Arch Venez Pueric Pediatr,* 2005;69:19-25.

Balzola F, et al. Panenteric IBD-like disease in a patient with regressive autism shown for the first time by wireless capsule enteroscopy: Another piece in the jig-saw of the gut-brain syndrome? *American Journal of Gastroenterology,* 2005. 100(4):979- 981.

Krigsman A, Boris M, Goldblatt A, Stott C. Clinical Presentation and Histologic Findings at Ileocolonoscopy in Children with Autistic Spectrum Disorder and Chronic Gastrointestinal Symptoms. *Autism Insights* 2009:1 1-11.

Balzola F, et al. Autistic enterocolitis: confirmation of a new inflammatory bowel disease in an Italian cohort of patients. *Gastroenterology.* 2005;128(Suppl. 2);A-303.

Galiatsatos P, et al. Autistic enterocolitis: fact or fiction. *Canadian Journal of Gastroenterology.* 2009;23:95-98.

[7] Demicheli V, Jefferson T, Rivetti A, et al. Vaccines for measles, mumps and rubella in children. *Cochrane Database Systematic Review,* 2005(4):CD004407. "The Cochrane Collaboration is an international, independent, not-for-profit organisation of over 27,000 contributors from more than 100 countries, dedicated to making up-to-date, accurate information about the effects of health care readily available worldwide." www.cochrane.org/

[8] The allegations, reported in theScientist.com (http://www.the-scientist.com/blog/display/55679/) involve the *Australasian Journal of Bone and Joint Medicine,* a publication paid for by pharmaceutical company Merck that amounted to a compendium of reprinted scientific articles and one-source reviews, most of which presented data favorable to Merck's

products. *The Scientist* obtained two 2003 issues of the journal — which bore the imprint of Elsevier's *Excerpta Medica* — neither of which carried a statement obviating Merck's sponsorship of the publication.

[9] Rout M. (2009, April 1). Vioxx maker Merck and Co drew up doctor hit list. Retrieved from http://aftermathnews.wordpress.com/2009/04/27/vioxx-maker-merck-and-co-drew-up-doctor-hit-list/

[10] Streicher ran the Sturmerverlag (Storm Trooper Publishing House). Streicher also published an introduction to the teacher's manual by Fritz Fink, *Die Judenfrage im Unterricht* [The Jewish Question in Classroom Instruction] (Nuremberg: Sturmerverlag, 1937). Excerpts from this teacher's manual can be found at: www.calvin.edu/academic/cas/gpa/fink.htm

[11] The Assessment and Qualifications Alliance is the largest of the three English exam boards.

[12] AQA Science (GCSE) 2006. Nelson Thornes (Publishers), p. 74.

[13] Emphasis added.

AFTERWORD

Ethics, Evidence and the Death of Medicine

Co-written with James Moody, Esq.*

First appeared in *The Autism File* magazine in April 2010.

Documents Prove Investigations of *The Lancet* Children Were Ethical

Acting on at least two false premises, the General Medical Council found *Dr. Wakefield and his colleagues guilty of performing research on children without ethics committee (EC) approval.

False premise 1.
The GMC confused diagnostic clinical tests with research.

False premise 2.
The GMC claimed there was no current EC approval that covered the research aspects of *The Lancet* paper. There was – the prosecution had failed in their duty to identify it.

The core finding by the General Medical Council against Dr. Wakefield and Professors Walker-Smith and Murch (*The Lancet* doctors) is that they performed unethical research on autistic children – children in whom they discovered a new bowel disease. Not to minimize the importance of ethics in medicine, the finding is of a "technical" violation because there was no finding that any child was harmed, only that for some children the diagnostic tests were not yet approved by the Royal Free's ethics committee. However, as shown in detail below, the documentary evidence demonstrates beyond all reasonable doubt that the diagnostic tests on *The Lancet* children were performed according to clinical need, that the research portion of the case series was approved by the EC, and that responsible officials at the Royal Free were well aware of the scope of the relevant approvals at the time and made no objection. At the same time, the GMC improperly reclassified routine clinical care as research and ignored pre-existing EC approval for research on bowel biopsies. The legacy of this trial threatens far more than *The Lancet* doctors, not only by denying autistic children the diagnostic tests and treatments they so desperately need but also by terrorizing doctors into depriving their patients of the innovative diagnostic and therapeutic interventions they deserve in favor of the relative safety of mediocrity in medicine.

Setting the Stage

Professor Sir Michael Rutter, the "dean" of UK autism experts, was the first to describe a case of vaccine-caused autism in the scientific literature in 1994. The UK Department of Health was largely responsible for fueling public doubt about MMR safety by introducing in 1988, and abruptly withdrawing in 1992, two MMR vaccines containing the Urabe AM-9 strain of mumps known to cause meningitis that had been withdrawn in Canada before its introduction in the UK. As a matter of fact, the US vaccine court began compensating for cases of vaccine-caused autism starting in 1991,[9] and the US Department of Health and Human Services has been secretly settling cases of vaccine-caused autism without a hearing also since 1991.[10] Clearly, vaccines can cause autism. What remains to be resolved is the body count, appropriate treatments, and reform of the vaccine schedule to prevent autism and other vaccine-caused chronic disorders. Nobody knows how much autism, or other chronic disorders, is caused by vaccines because no comprehensive scientific studies have ever been done comparing the health of unvaccinated children to those fully vaccinated. Some are of the opinion that because they fear accountability and liability, public health authorities are now actively opposing such research. However, this research is absolutely necessary to prevent disease and maintain public confidence in vaccines.

Why then does Dr. Wakefield get all the attention, blame, or credit (depending on your perspective) for simply posing the hypothesis of a possible association between MMR and autism and calling for further research? Unlike others who ran for cover, he continues to undertake a program of careful scientific research designed to determine how many children have been affected. He is looking for the precise mechanisms and markers for this type of vaccine injury because his goals are preventing avoidable vaccine injury, treating those already injured, and of restored public trust. The most visible of Dr. Wakefield's early work was a paper published in the February 1998 issue of *The Lancet* reporting a case series of 12 children who developed autism and bowel disease, the majority following MMR vaccination. The paper cautiously warned that no causal association was shown and called for further research. This commenced the political war to suppress vaccine safety science and to cover up the denial of appropriate treatment to autistic children who might be victims of vaccine injury. The GMC investigation of *The Lancet* doctors, begun in 2004 and extending into the year 2010, is just the most recent field of battle in this titanic struggle. The initial GMC findings, released January 28, 2010, were predictably followed by *Lancet* editor Horton's formal withdrawal of the case series, citing ethical concerns. Horton had described the paper in his GMC testimony as "important new information that would be of interest to a general medical readership." But now, because he's at the eye of this political storm over vaccine safety, he has committed "editorial genocide," attempting to erase the contribution of these 12 children.

Research vs. Clinical Practice

Approval by any hospital's ethics committee is, of course, a prerequisite to conducting research on patients, but no such oversight or approval is required for ordinary clinical practice. EC approval was an obvious, routine, and clearly understood procedure, especially at teaching hospitals like the Royal Free, long before the mid-1990s. Since the consequences of doing unapproved research on patients can obviously be serious, doctors must have an easy way to determine where diagnostic and clinical care ends and research begins. Diagnostic testing and clinical care are primarily for the benefit of the particular patient; research, on the other hand, is a systematic investigation, an "experimental study," designed to contribute to generalizable knowledge. GMC ethics guidance specifically exempts "innovative therapeutic interventions designed to benefit individual patients" from "research" requiring EC approval.

The authoritative Belmont Report recognized that the precise boundaries between clinical practice and research (requiring ethics oversight for the protection of human subjects) are "blurred" because—in practice they often occur together. The term "practice" refers to "interventions that are designed solely to enhance the well-being of an individual patient or client and that have a reasonable expectation of success. The purpose of medical or behavioral practice is to provide diagnosis, preventive treatment, or therapy to particular individuals." The fact that some forms of practice have elements other than immediate benefit to the individual, however, should not confuse the general distinction between research and practice. Even when a procedure applied in practice may benefit some other person, it remains an intervention designed to enhance the well-being of a particular individual or groups of individuals; thus, it is clinical practice and need not be reviewed as research. The guiding principle in the practice of medicine is the primacy of patient care. In the service of this overarching goal, the defining characteristic of clinical diagnosis is the definition of the disease entity, even when no immediate treatment is possible. The Belmont Report continues: "When a clinician departs in a significant way from standard or accepted practice, the innovation does not, in and of itself, constitute research. The fact that a procedure is 'experimental,' in the sense of new, untested or different, does not automatically place it in the category of research. Radically new procedures of this description should, however, be made the object of formal research at an early stage in order to determine whether they are safe and effective." In other words, introducing innovative interventions for the clinical purpose of benefiting the specific children being evaluated is not research, even if data about the intervention is collected from medical records for research purposes in a retrospective or prospective manner.

Diagnostic Tests Appropriate to Clinical Need

The children reported in *The Lancet* were all sick. All had a history of normal or near normal development followed by loss of acquired skills (regression). All had gut issues, which was why they were referred to the world leader in the field of pediatric gastroenterology, Professor John Walker-Smith. At that time, each child's local National Health Service Trust had to pay for care, so the "extra-contractual referral" had to be locally approved and justified by the clinical needs of each child to be seen at a tertiary care facility such as the Royal Free. Diagnostic testing was justified by each child's medical history and clinical presentation. Such diagnostic investigations, indicated by clinical need, did not require EC approval because they were undertaken in the patient's interest for the purpose of **establishing a diagnosis** and **directing treatment**. These diagnostic investigations included colonoscopies to look at the children's bowel for treatable inflammation, while some had lumbar punctures to look at the cerebrospinal fluid, principally for evidence of mitochondrial dysfunction.[1] Both are routine tests for children with unexplained symptoms of intestinal and/or neurological dysfunction. The clinical imperative for investigations such as colonoscopy and lumbar puncture in the autistic children was stated explicitly by all three doctors in evidence at the GMC hearing, and it was contained in a succession of contemporaneous documents from 1996 onwards, examples of which are provided below.

EC Approval for Biopsy Research

On September 5, 1995, Professor Walker-Smith was granted generic EC approval for biopsy research on children undergoing diagnostic colonoscopy for bowel symptoms (designated by the EC as project 162-95).[2] The consent form for two extra biopsies signed by parents explained that "chronic inflammatory bowel diseases are still little understood and their cause is unknown. It is therefore of great value for laboratory research to have such biopsies available to study how inflammation in the bowel develops and is influenced by treatment... Whether or not you agree to this will in no way influence your assessment or treatment."

Children with a pervasive developmental disorder and severe bowel disease started coming to the Royal Free Hospital for clinical investigation beginning in mid-1996. The first 12 of these consecutively referred children were reported as *The Lancet* case series. The only aspect of "research" involving these children was the collection of the two additional biopsies and the later biopsy analysis in the laboratory, approved as EC 162-95. All the children had the EC-approved research consent form included in their files, as well as consents for other clinical procedures.

Based upon common features reported in this initial group of children (termed a "pilot study"), the Royal Free team developed a detailed clinical and research protocol that included research aspects in addition to the previously approved biopsies such as genetic testing and markers of brain inflammation. The majority of these additional research tests were to be undertaken on samples left over from the diagnostic tests. The application to the EC was submitted on September 16, 1996, designated as project 172-96, and approved on December 18, 1996. EC approval required that children enrolled in this research study be given an information sheet and that a signed a consent form be placed in each child's file.

None of *The Lancet* Children Were Part of the EC 172-96 Research Project

The EC 172-96 handout to parents began with the title of the study, "A New Paediatric Syndrome: Enteritis and Disintegrative Disorder Following Measles/Rubella Vaccination," and explained that the Royal Free team "have formulated the hypothesis that in certain (perhaps genetically susceptible) children, live-virus vaccines may produce long-term inflammation of the intestine and failure to absorb, in particular, vitamin B12... We would like to carry out a series of tests which, we believe, will help us to establish the features of this possible disease. Our aim is to characterize the problem so that, for the future, we may be able to treat affected children and improve their wellbeing." The consent form stated: "I have read and understood the aims and nature of this study, and have discussed in detail, the implications of the study with the Doctors concerned. I hereby agree to let my child _____ take part in the study. I understand that I can withdraw my child from the study at any stage without prejudicing his/her management or treatment in any way." None of *The Lancet* children had these papers in their file.

The fact that the files of *The Lancet* children all contained the 162-96 EC consent for research biopsies and neither the EC-approved information sheet for the 172-96 research study nor the associated consent form makes confusion impossible. The GMC allegation and finding that *The Lancet* children were enrolled in EC project 172-95 is objectively impossible as shown by the consent forms in each child's record.

The EC Knew *The Lancet* Children Were Being Seen for Clinical Need, Not Research
Crucially, the application submitted to the EC for 172-96 explained that the diagnostic tests were for clinical purposes. The EC application asked: "Would the procedure(s) or sample(s) be taken especially for this investigation or as part of normal patient care?" Our answer was:

> *Yes: in view of the symptoms and signs manifested by these patients, **all of the procedures and the majority of the samples are clinically indicated**[8] [i.e., normal patient care]. Additional intestinal biopsies (5 per patient) will be taken for viral analysis. DNA for genotyping will use blood cells isolated from the routine blood sample and will not require an additional sample.*

The EC obviously contemplated a situation such as this where the tests included in the investigative protocol included both those for clinical and research purposes. If the EC believed that the diagnostic testing described in the application was not appropriate for the children with the indicated symptoms, then surely a question would have been raised. So, the following question arises: Why isn't the GMC prosecuting EC chair Dr. Pegg and the other members of the EC for approving such supposedly risky and reckless procedures?

Children with bowel disease and PDD kept being referred to the Royal Free while the formal protocol was pending before the EC. They continued to receive diagnostic tests and clinical care appropriate to children exhibiting symptoms of bowel disease and loss of acquired developmental skills. However, straightforward clinical and ethics issues had by this time already become hotly "political" because the topic of the proposed research included possible vaccine damage and were thus receiving careful scrutiny. In response to an inquiry about the testing done on these children, Professor Walker-Smith explained in a November 11, 1996, letter to EC chairman Pegg that

> *These children suffer from a disease with a "hopeless prognosis" in relation to their cerebral disintegrative disorder. They have often not had the level of investigation which we would regard as adequate for a child presenting with such a devastating condition. In relation to their gastrointestinal symptoms which will be present in all the children we investigate, these have often been under-investigated.*[3]

He explained that each child <u>already being treated</u> was certain to receive "reasonable benefit," the key requirement distinguishing clinical practice from research, by

> *a. Establishing a diagnosis and excluding metabolic and other causes*
>
> *b. Commencing on a therapeutic regime.*

The clinical benefit to each of *The Lancet* children clearly distinguishes that case series from research. Professor Walker-Smith confirmed, beyond doubt, that children had already been investigated well before EC approval for project 172-96 was given:

> *We have so far investigated 5 such children on a **clinical need basis**,[8] all in fact have proved to have evidence of chronic bowel inflammation. … I can confirm that children would have these investigations even if there were no trial. I must make it clear that we would not be investigating children without gastrointestinal symptoms.*

It would have been unethical, if not appalling, to have refused care and turned these children away while the EC was reviewing the prospective research protocol.

Dr. Wakefield again notified the EC on February 3, 1997, that additional children had been seen in the clinic prior to starting the 176-96 research project. He wrote to amend the proposed protocol by deleting the MRI and EEG in light of the fact that neurological studies had not revealed any helpful clinical information, and adding an intestinal permeability test.[4] Deletion of the MRI and EEG was purely a clinical decision taken by Walker-Smith in the children's best interests, i.e., <u>not research</u>, but was mentioned since Pegg wished to be informed of "any" changes. In this letter Wakefield confirmed that, in addition to the 5 children referred to by Walker-Smith in his November 11 letter, a further 4 children had been investigated, and now a total of 8 children had evidence of intestinal inflammation. Thus the EC knew in February 1997 that 9 children – 9 of the 12 who went on to be reported in *The Lancet* – had already been seen and evaluated in the clinic, but those children had nothing to do with project 172-96. It should have been evident to Dr. Pegg that this protocol was still being revised based on what was learned from the pilot study.

Ultimately and ironically, project 172-96 was never undertaken. Funding for the additional research elements contained in this proposal was not forthcoming, and it was not pursued further. *The Lancet* doctors, therefore, did not violate the EC approval for 172-96 by enrolling children who did not meet the inclusion criteria and did not perform "research" on these children before the project's start date—because research project 172-96 was never started.

On the other hand, the biopsy research covered by 162-95 proved to be extremely informative, and this is where Dr. Wakefield's and Professor Murch's research focused. Professor Walker-Smith wrote again to Pegg on July 15, 1998:

> *Further to our original study [The Lancet case series], we are now continuing to see such children by clinical need and performing ileo-colonoscopy and limited blood tests in order to decide whether to give such children Mesalazine [anti-inflammatory medication for inflammatory bowel disease]. As Dr. Wakefield is carefully analyzing our results and some of the biopsies being taken are being used for research (we already have research permission for taking extra biopsies in children who we colonoscope). I would like formally to request Ethical Committee approval for our clinical research analysis of these children who we are continuing to see by clinical need.[5]*

He requested only continued permission to analyze the results of the clinical data for the purposes of publication and this was granted. The whole matter was reviewed by the dean of the medical school, Professor Zuckerman, on July 15, 1998, whose annotated approval read:

> *All the necessary steps with Ethical Committee and other matters.*

High-Level Oversight Without Objection to the Clinical Care
Further evidence of the level of intense scrutiny given to the appropriateness of the clinical care of *The Lancet* children comes from a July 6, 1998, letter from Professor Sir David Hull ex-chairman of the Joint Committee on Vaccination and Immunization—clearly aware that vaccine safety research was underway and concerned about potential government liability—to Dean Zuckerman seeking his help "on a matter of personal concern." Hull was concerned that "many more children had been similarly investigated and still more were on the waiting list." Referencing the Hull letter, Professor Walker-Smith again reassured Dean Zuckerman in his July 14, 1998, letter that "[t]hese subsequent children are being seen by clinical need to decide upon a treatment and help these children."

Also in response to the Hull letter, Professor Walker-Smith wrote to Royal Free CEO Martin Else explaining:

> *The children with autism who have gastrointestinal symptoms, from the very beginning, have been investigated according to clinical need. This has been approved by the Ethics Committee. Also it is routine for us to have ethical approval to take endoscopic biopsies for research purposes with parental consent for all children who are endoscoped. We have never moved outside any frame that has not been approved by the Ethics Committee or indeed that is outside the bounds of ethical behaviour in the widest sense. We have the clearest evidence both published and unpublished that these children have a form of chronic inflammatory bowel disease... The children that we are seeing with autism and gastrointestinal symptoms deserve the kind of investigation that we are performing.*

Again referencing the Hull letter, Pegg wrote to Zuckerman on July 24, 1998, explaining:

> *We approved data collection from clinically indicated investigations. It is not, at present, the role of an ethics committee to question clinicians' judgment as to what are and what are not clinically indicated investigations. However, we do not just take the word of*

the investigator, rather we ask for independent expert review of all applications. In this case Dr. Owen Epstein provided a review of the project and I have a letter from him "strongly supporting" the study.

Dean Zuckerman wrote back to Sir David Hull on July 28, 1998, assuring him that all of the children were seen according to clinical need and that oversight by the EC was appropriate. With all this scrutiny, at the highest levels, where was the objection by anybody that the diagnostic tests performed on *The Lancet* children were somehow unethical?

The GMC Improperly Reclassified Clinical Care as Research

There were no ethical violations in relation to the investigation and reporting of *The Lancet* 12. No child was subjected to any invasive test for the purpose of research. The GMC prosecution rested on the claim that *The Lancet* children were part of research project 172-96. It appears to have concealed EC 162-95 research approval for biopsies, and, for the first time, attempted to second-guess the judgment of eminent clinicians about what investigations were clinically indicated to diagnose and treat desperately ill children.

The GMC did not find Professor Walker-Smith, the senior clinician, guilty of dishonesty. The panel must have accepted the integrity of his position on the clinical merits of these tests both in 1996 and now. The documents confirm not only this doctor's position on the clinical need for investigation and the inadequacy of previous investigations on these children, but make it clear that the Royal Free EC, the dean, the CEO, and even Sir David Hull knew all along that autistic children with bowel disease were being seen and investigated according to clinical need. In 1996-98 senior medical staff knew what was being done and what approval was in place.

GMC Complainant Brian Deer Knew the Biopsy Research Was Approved by the Ethics Committee

Documents recently released under the Freedom of Information Act (FOIA) reveal that the complainant, journalist Brian Deer, knew in 2004 that the research biopsies had EC approval as part of 162-95. This was disclosed to him in January 2004 through his FOIA request to the Strategic Health Authority that has responsibility for the Royal Free Hospital.[6]

You may think it strange that although this document was clearly relevant to the conduct of research on biopsies taken from children under the care of Professor Walker-Smith, the GMC appeared to know nothing of it. Presumably Deer disclosed this document to the GMC, otherwise he would have risked exposure as a fraud for withholding key evidence following any serious initial investigation by GMC staff. It was not included in the documents upon which the GMC relied in formulating their original charges against the doctors that had been supplied by Deer with his complaint. Nor was it ever disclosed in the documents supplied to the defendants by the GMC, including all of the unused material that the GMC is obliged to disclose. In fact, the GMC's findings explicitly stated:

> The research study was carried out on Child "x" without the approval of the Ethics Committee in that it was not research covered by any Ethics Committee application other than that for Project 172-96.

Deer either concealed this information from the prosecution, or the prosecution concealed it from the doctors. In the light of the EC's prior approval of biopsy research in 162-95, Deer's 2004 allegation of unethical research would have been rendered palpably false. Whether or not Deer disclosed this key document, a competent investigation by the GMC should have revealed it. Since the approval documents for 162-95 were in the possession of the Royal Free's ethics committee, they should have been obtained by the GMC's lawyers and volunteered by Dr. Pegg, the committee's chairman, during the process of taking his witness statement. There is no evidence in any of the GMC material that this ever happened, which must raise a serious question over prosecutorial competence, if not misconduct. Moreover, EC chairman Pegg made no mention of this approval in his statement or evidence, implicating him as well.

The prosecution proceeded on the basis of a preconceived assumption of guilt rather than conducting a fair and thorough investigation. Perhaps this whole GMC case has not been an honest effort to protect patients but politically motivated scapegoating after all? As *Lancet* editor Horton boasted in his 2004 book *MMR: Science and Fiction,*

> The GMC seemed nonplussed by Reid's (the then Health Secretary) intervention urging the GMC to investigate Wakefield as a matter of urgency. In truth they had not a clue where to begin. At a dinner I attended on 23 February 2004, one medical regulator and I discussed the Wakefield case. He seemed unsure of how the Council could play a useful part in resolving any confusion. As we talked over coffee

while the other dinner guests were departing, he scribbled down some possible lines of investigation and passed me his card, suggesting that I contact him directly if anything else came to mind. He seemed keen to pursue Wakefield, especially given ministerial interest. Here was professionally led regulation of doctors in action--notes exchanged over liqueurs in a beautifully wood-paneled room of one of medicine's most venerable institutions.

Perhaps this is just one part of an ongoing campaign to stop research into the safety of MMR and vaccines on the one hand, and on the other to conceal the appalling refusal of the NHS to provide proper care for autistic children with severe GI problems, which is itself an egregious violation of basic medical ethics.

So it was that *The Lancet* case series had the appropriate ethical approval for the biopsy research and this ethical approval was stated in the paper as published. If Deer provided the GMC with evidence of 162-95, then the prosecution withheld the details of this EC approval from the panel.

While Dr. Wakefield's research had operated under 162-95, the documents were not in his possession but that of the ethics committee. During his evidence Dr. Wakefield stressed the importance of relying, not on memory, but on the original documents, many of which—like 162-95—only belatedly came to light during the oral evidence. Wherever possible, he had avoided speculation during the preparation of the defense on the basis that reconstruction of the events of 9 years earlier, in the absence of the contemporaneous documents, was fraught with hazard. He was right. The GMC's failure to either obtain or disclose crucial documents such as 162-95 had, ironically, damned the defendants' chance of a fair trial. The GMC lawyers may claim in mitigation that, in applying the wrong ethical approval to *The Lancet* study, they had relied upon an erroneous statement made by Professor Murch in 2004, a statement prepared hastily, under great duress, and crucially, in the absence of the relevant documents. This point was made repeatedly by the defense during the hearing; it fell on deaf ears.

The GMC Panel's comment on the crucial matter of prior valid ethical approval was as dismissive as it was insipid, and utterly bereft of any analysis:

The Panel has heard that ethical approval had been sought and granted for other trials and it has been specifically suggested that Project 172-

96 was never undertaken and that in fact, The Lancet 12 children's investigations were clinically indicated and the research parts of those clinically justified investigations were covered by Project 162-95. In the light of all the available evidence, the Panel rejected this proposition.[7]

Dire Implications

The GMC findings have dire consequences for the practice of medicine generally, necessary treatments for desperately ill autistic children, and for the future of the GMC in its role of protecting patients. January 28, 2010, may go down as the day that innovative clinical care died in the UK, killed off by the post hoc reclassification of such care as unethical research. Imagine bringing your desperately ill child to a clinic, only be told by the most eminent doctors in the field that their hands are tied, and they can do nothing because the condition and treatments have not yet been well described in the medical literature, and they have to design a "research" protocol, submit it to a committee, and wait months for approval. Preposterous? Of course, but this is what will happen if the GMC findings lead to any sort of punitive action. Doctors just won't take the risk of a protracted investigation that may be for collateral purposes such as the settling of scores, much less of losing their license, and will settle in to the safe mediocrity of doling out medicine "by the books." Medicine will no longer be a learned profession but just a series of rote steps performed mechanically and utterly without inspiration. Patients' care will suffer, which is exactly the opposite of GMC's supposed mission. Although all of medicine will suffer, the impact will be most immediately borne by the most severely ill autistic children. They will continue to be denied the diagnosis and care that is their basic human and ethical right. The GMC has become complicit in this phase of the overall battle to get at the scientific truth about vaccines and autism, and other chronic disorders, sacrificing these children on an altar made of deliberate ignorance of the preventable harm from vaccines and indifference to their medical needs. If we are to retain the benefits of vaccines, we must fulfill our duty to these children and to the doctors brave enough to come to their aid.

Doctors beware: prepare to be second-guessed by medical regulators on your clinical judgment and specifically on whether—despite your training, expertise, and documentary evidence—tests you undertake on the sickest of your patients are clinically indicated or for the purpose of research.

Endnotes

[1] Based on the clinical protocol for children undergoing neurological deterioration form Birmingham Children's Hospital.

[2] Ethical Practices Committee approval for taking of research biopsies during colonoscopy EPC 162-95.

[3] Letter, John Walker-Smith to Dr. Michael Pegg, Nov. 11, 1996.

[4] Letter, Dr. Wakefield to Dr. Pegg, Feb. 3, 1997.

[5] Letter, JWS to Dr. Pegg, July 15, 1998. Copies to Zuckerman and annotated July 17, 1998.

[6] Letter from John Walker-Smith to Ms. Carroll of the Royal Free Ethical Practices Committee Feb. 27, 1997.

[7] Fitness to Practise Panel applying the General Medical Council's Preliminary Proceedings Committee and Professional Conduct Committee (Procedure) Rules 1988. Finding on facts. Jan. 28, 2010.

[8] Emphasis added.

[9] Age of Autism. (2009, February 27). Why is the Media Ignoring the Bailey Banks Autism Vaccine Decision? Retrieved from http://www.ageofautism.com/2009/02/why-is-the-mediaignoring-the-bailey-banks-autism-vaccine-decision.html.

See also Bailey Banks, by his father Kenneth Banks v. Secretary of the Department of Health and Human Services. United States Court of Federal Claims. 20 July 2007.

Retrieved from http://www.uscfc.uscourts.gov/sites/default/files/Abell.BANKS.02-0738V.pdf

[10] Attkisson S. (2008, June 19). Vaccine Watch. CBS News Investigates: Primary Source. Retrieved from http://www.cbsnews.com/8301-501263_162-4194102-501263.html.

Epilogue

There is more to come – much more: the journeys of fellow travelers, another whistleblower, misconduct in Congress, and an over-the-counter nutritional supplement called transfer factor, a naturally occurring substance, intended as an immune-enhancing agent to help children clear measles infection but branded falsely as an MMR vaccine "competitor." Despite a lack of evidence, it has been alleged that I started a child on transfer factor. In fact, the parents chose to use this non-prescription supplement for their child. It was never used by me or my colleagues as an "experimental drug," and the issue of pediatric qualifications was entirely irrelevant. And so on…

As I share some final thoughts, rumors of a possible $2M fraud (and CDC collusion) by Dr. Paul Thorsen (a senior investigator on the famously "negative" Madsen Danish studies that claimed, wrongly, to exonerate a role for thimerosal and MMR in autism[1]) abound. Further rumors indicate that another government witness in US vaccine court and reputed autism expert is under investigation for ethical violations in Canada. In the UK, Rutter, Horton, Zuckerman, Pegg, and Salisbury are the subjects of complaints to the GMC. Oh, yes, and another several thousand children have gone to the wall while this "Theatre of the Absurd" has been playing out. Deaths,[2] deportation,[3] imprisonment,[4] and suicide[5] – will these too turn out to be avoidable adverse vaccine reactions?

Stop for a moment. Politicians, regulators, manufacturers, attorneys, bloggers, and hangers-on: Act now to protect children. Act now to protect the benefits of the vaccine program. Put **safety first** above any other consideration. Insist on this, Mr. and Mrs. Gates.

There is no place for indulging futile displacement activity, sanctimonious posturing, and self-protectionism. In the battle for the hearts and minds of the public, you have already lost… Why? Because the parents are right; their stories are true; their children's brains are damaged; there is a major, major problem. In the US, increasingly coercive vaccine mandates and fear-mongering advertising campaigns are a measure of your failure – vaccine uptake is not a reflection of public confidence, but of these coercive measures, and without public confidence, you have nothing.

With the issue of vaccine safety in mind, in 2001 I got together with Dr. Laura Hewitson, an outstanding researcher, at that time at the University of Pittsburgh. With colleagues, we designed a study that should have been done many years before. We set out to examine the safety of the US vaccine schedule – starting with the hepatitis B vaccine (HBV) given on day one of life through to pre-school boosters. The first paper – the first of many – reported delayed acquisition of survival reflexes (e.g., feeding) in infant monkeys after the day one HBV shot (containing mercury preservative). Following rigorous peer-review and online publication in *Neurotoxicology*, the paper was withdrawn, not apparently, on the instructions of the scientific editor, but by the publishing company Elsevier.[6] The links between this company and the pharmaceutical industry have been reported by Mark Blaxill in one of his excellent pieces for *Age of Autism*.[6] Science, it would seem, is available to the highest bidder.

Emperor Nero did not fiddle while Rome burned, but he did blame the fire on others – the Christians – whom he put to the sword to appease the angry mob. Governments, in contrast with Nero, are guilty of both – they have fiddled and appeased. It will be left to future generations to repair and rebuild.

There will be victory of a sort. And it will be a victory from the bottom up; in the true spirit of the American Constitution, the people will have their say. It will not come from the top down because a phalanx of lobbyists, "experts," and true believers stands between the President and the people he is sworn to serve.

Sinking slow, out over Crystal Mountain, the Texan sun still hurts the land. The cedars draw on parched earth. And the sun is gone. Stars creep into the night sky and the forest begins to move. My children are asleep and my beer is cold. From the lips of Willie Nelson, the ballad of Bobby McGee falls with a salty melancholy: *"I'd trade all my tomorrows for a single yesterday."* And for a moment I am there, on the cold, wet precipice of Hounds Ghyll viaduct, 180 feet above oblivion as the small boy looks questioningly into my face, slips my hand, and is gone.

Endnotes

[1] Wakefield AJ, Blaxill M, Stott C. MMR and Autism in Perspective: the Denmark Story. *Journal of American Physicians and Surgeons.* 2004;9(3):89-91.

[2] Marikar S, Childs D, Chitale R. (2009, January 5). Death Certificate: John Travolta's Son Died of a Seizure. Retrieved from http://abcnews.go.com/Entertainment/ MindMoodNews/story?id=6576215&page=1.

[3] Campsie A. (2009, July 16). Deportation of Hacker to US for trial would be 'disastrous'. *The Herald.* Retrieved from http://www.heraldscotland.com/deportation-of-hacker-to-us-for-trial-would-be-disastrous-1.914708.

[4] Information for criminal justice professionals (n.d.) Retrived from http://www.nas.org. uk/nas/jsp/polopoly.jsp?d=471.

[5] National suicide prevention strategy for England. (n.d.) Retrieved from http://www. nas.org.uk/nas/jsp/polopoly.jsp?d=2520&a=2371.

[6] Blaxill M. (2010, March 2). Joan Cranmer's Fateful Decisions and the Suppression of Autism Science. *Age of Autism.* Retrieved from http://www.ageofautism.com/2010/03/ joan-cranmers-fateful-decisions-and-the-suppression-of-autism-science.html#more.

Date	Events at the Royal Free	Events at the UK Department of Health	Events at The Lancet	Relevant scientific publications other than from Royal Free	Events in the national media	Events at the GMC
1971				Chess reports autism following congenital rubella infection[1]		
1975				Rivinus et al. report autistic spectrum disorder after brain inflammation caused by measles virus[2]		
1979		*Trivirix* MMR vaccine containing dangerous mumps strain Urabe AM-9, licensed in Canada.		Deykin and MacMahon link measles and mumps exposures to autism[3]		
1986		Cases of mumps **meningitis** from MMR vaccine reported in Canada.[4]				
1987		MMR vaccine planned for UK. Dr. Salisbury responsible for "Strategy design and policy implementation"[5]				

[1] Chess S. Autism in children with congenital rubella. *J Autism Dev Disord.* 1971;1:33-47.
[2] Rivinus TM, Jamison DL, and Graham PJ. Childhood organic neurological disease presenting as psychiatric disorder. *Arch Dis Child.* 1975;50:115-119.
[3] Deykin EY and MacMahon B. Viral exposure and autism. *American Journal of Epidemiology.* 1979;109:628-638.
[4] Champagne et al. *Can Dis Weekly Rep.* 1987;13:155-157.
[5] Curriculum vitae of Dr. Salisbury.

Date				
November 23, 1987		Distribution of MMR in Canada officially suspended [Bureau of Biologics].		
March 1988	AW starts work at Royal Free at around this time	**Anaphylaxis** noted by the Joint Committee on Vaccination and Immunization (JCVI) to be a serious and potentially fatal complication of measles-containing vaccines.		
July 1988		Product recall of MMR (*Trivirix*) in Ontario		
July 1988		*Trivirix* re-branded as *Pluserix*[6] is licensed in UK against advice of Whistleblower.		
1989		JCVI, aware of meningitis cases in Canada, UK, and Japan, takes no action to withdraw vaccine or warn parents.	Cases of meningitis appear in UK soon after MMR introduced. Reported in *The Lancet*.[7]	Cases of meningitis after Urabe MMR reported in Japan.[8]
September 18, 1989		Second brand of Urabe-containing MMR licensed in UK (*Immravax*, Pasteur Merieux; later Aventis Pasteur). No mention of meningitis risk in *Immravax* product license.[9]		

[6] *Trivirix* and *Pluserix* contain Measles [Schwarz; minimum of 1000 TCID50], Mumps [Urabe; 20,000 TCID50], Rubella [RA 27/3; 1000 TCID50]
[7] Mumps meningitis following measles, mumps, and rubella immunisation [letter]. *The Lancet*, vol. 2, July 8, 1989, p. 98; comments in vol. 2, August 12, 1989, pp. 394-5; vol. 2, September 16, 1989, p. 677.
[8] Nakatani H, et al. Development of Vaccination Policy in Japan: Current Issues and Policy Directions. *Jpn. J. Infect. Dis.* 2002;55:101-111. Retrieved from www.nih_go.jp/JJID/55/101/pdf.
[9] Product Licence No. 6745/0020. Granted 18th Sept 1989.7d.

Date	Events at the Royal Free	Events at the UK Department of Health	Events at The Lancet	Relevant scientific publications other than from Royal Free	Events in the national media	Events at the GMC
May 4, 1990		JCVI minutes on Japan: "Of especial concern to the ARVI [Committee on Adverse Reactions to Vaccination and Immunisation] were reports of a high level of meningoencephalitis [inflammation of brain and its coverings] associated with administration of MMR." JCVI dismisses concerns.				
1990		*Trivirix* license revoked in Canada, followed by Malaysia, Philippines, Singapore. MMR secretly withdrawn in Australia.				
September 17, 1990		JCVI minutes indicate more cases of meningitis cases following MMR reported in UK. Rate much higher than that detected by the adverse reactions reporting system in place. JCVI takes no action to withdraw vaccine or warn parents.				
1991-1992		**MMR scare starts:** "…in 1991/92 it [the Legal Aid Board] first began to receive an increasing number of applications on behalf of children, claiming personal injury as a result of the MMR/MR vaccination."[10]				

[10] Letter from Legal Services Commission (formerly LAB) to Brian Deer under Freedom of Information Act. December 22, 2006.
[Note: MR Vaccine had not been used at this stage, so these claims must relate to MMR.]

October 2, 1992	AW first writes to Dr. Salisbury warning of concerns over measles and Crohn's disease, requesting a meeting and raising issue of research funding. No meeting arranged.			
July 1991	UK safety study of MMR and meningitis 4 years after vaccine was licensed. Results showed much higher incidence than detected by existing surveillance method.			
September 11, 1992	SmithKline Beecham issues urgent stop to *Pluserix* use in UK.			
September 15, 1992	Suspension of *Pluserix* and *Immravax* in UK and replacement with MMR II (Merck, Sharp & Dohme)			*Telegraph* newspaper "Brain Disease Ban on Vaccine." Peter Ballot announces withdrawal of *Pluserix* and *Immravax* one week before DoH was due to tell doctors.[11]

[11] Telegraph cuttings library system, cwlib2.8080/telegraph/cls

Date	Events at the Royal Free	Events at the UK Department of Health	Events at The Lancet	Relevant scientific publications other than from Royal Free	Events in the national media	Events at the GMC
September 15, 1992					*Evening Standard.* Lord Ashley (former MP Jack Ashley) states: "The government had first known of this problem in March last year (18 months previously) when Health Minister Virginia Bottomeley wrote saying that the vaccine was being investigated due to reports of serious problems."[27]	
September 16, 1992					*The Independent* newspaper reports: "Children received vaccine despite meningitis link."[12]	
1992				High risk of **anaphylaxis** after re-vaccination reported in US.[13]		

[12] Hall C. (1992, September 16). Children received vaccine despite meningitis link. *The Independent.* Retrieved from http://www.independent.co.uk/news/uk/children-received-vaccine-despite-meningitis-link-1551697.html

[13] Kaler A, Berger DK, Bateman WB, Dubitsky J, Covitz K. Allergic reactions to MMR vaccine. *Pediatrics.* 1992;89:168-9.

[27] Harper M. (1992, September 15). Government is accused on baby vaccine danger. *Evening Standard.* See also: http://www.publications.parliament.uk/pa/cm199192/cmhansrd/1992-03-02/Writtens-2.html

January 1993	AW writes again to Salisbury expressing concerns over vaccine safety and requests a meeting. No meeting arranged.			
1994		Rutter publishes paper linking vaccines to autism.[14]		
October 14, 1994	AW writes to Dr. Aylsa Baxter of SmithKline Beecham to alert her to safety concerns. AW requests meeting.			
October 1994	AW writes again to Salisbury expressing concerns about revaccination campaign and urging a meeting. Letter copied to Minister of Health. Meeting arranged for *after* revaccination campaign (see below).			
November 1994	UK Measles Rubella mass revaccination campaign aimed at all school children. Parents not warned of anaphylaxis risk.			

[14] Rutter et al. Autism and known medical conditions; myth and substance. J. Child Psychol. Psychol. Psychiat. 1994;35:311-322.

Date	Events at the Royal Free	Events at the UK Department of Health	Events at The Lancet	Relevant scientific publications other than from Royal Free	Events in the national media	Events at the GMC
January 10, 1995		First meeting between AW and DoH.				
April 28, 1995	Publication by The Lancet of possible link between measles vaccine and inflammatory bowel disease.[15]					
May 19, 1995	Initial contact from parents of children with regressive autism – Rosemary Kessick (mother to Child 2 of The Lancet 12)					
June 29, 1995	Child 2 referred to Professor John Walker-Smith (JWS) at St. Bartholomew's Hospital.			Plesner from Denmark reports onset of gait disturbance (ataxia) specifically after MMR.[16]		
September 5, 1995	JWS transfers to the Royal Free Hospital and is granted ethics committee approval 162-95 for biopsy research on children undergoing ileo-colonoscopy.					

[15] Thompson NP, et al. Is measles vaccination a risk factor for inflammatory bowel disease? The Lancet 1995; 345:1071-1074.

[16] Plesner AM. Gait disturbances after measles mumps rubella vaccine. The Lancet 1995;345:316.

Date	Event
December 17, 1995	*The Sunday Times* reports AW's work on measles vaccine and inflammatory bowel disease and Dr. Reed Warren's investigation of MMR and autism in US.[17]
January 1996	AW meeting with lawyer Richard Barr and agreement to act as expert in vaccine/Crohn's disease litigation.
January - September 1996	Preparation of clinical (JWS) and research (AW) protocol for investigation of children with developmental disorder and intestinal symptoms.
July 1996	First child of *The Lancet 12* attends Royal Free Hospital.
August 1996	Funding for LAB pilot study for measles virus detection in five children with Crohn's and five with autism and bowel disease approved. Funding placed in suspense account by Zuckerman, Dean of Royal Free School of Medicine.

[17] Roberts Y. (1995, December 17). A Shot in the Dark. *Sunday Times Magazine*, pp. 17-23.

Date	Events at the Royal Free	Events at the UK Department of Health	Events at The Lancet	Relevant scientific publications other than from Royal Free	Events in the national media	Events at the GMC
September 1996	Clinical and research protocol 172-96 submitted to Royal Free ethics committee for consideration for approval of research elements.					
October 1996	Dean of medical school comes under pressure from the UK government to stop vaccine safety research.					
October 11, 1996	Dean writes to ethics committee of the British Medical Association (BMA) over the ethics of the LAB pilot study.					
November 27, 1996					*The Independent* newspaper prints **"Law: A shot in the Dark"**: "William is one of 10 children taking part in **a pilot study** at the **Royal Free Hospital** in London which is investigating possible links between the measles vaccine with the bowel disorder	

Date		
November 27, 1996	Crohn's disease and with autism. This study is being organized by Norfolk Solicitors Dawbarns".[18]	
January 7, 1997	Ethics committee approval given for larger study of 25 children with developmental disorder (172-96).	
January 9, 1997	AW writes to chairman of ethics committee (Pegg) to report results of pilot study (The Lancet 12) and indicate protocol modifications to 172-96.	
January 21, 1997	Meeting between AW and colleagues to discuss AW's role in litigation followed by written explanation.	
January 1997	Last child of The Lancet 12 investigated at Royal Free. Many more children continued then to be seen.	
February 10, 1997	Meeting at Royal Free with members of JCVI at AW's request to alert them to MMR-autism issue.	Ring, et al. link measles infection to autism in Israel.[19]

[18] Langdon-Down G. (1996. November 27). "Law: A shot in the Dark." *The Independent.* Page 25.
[19] Ring A, Barak Y, Ticher A. Evidence for an infectious aetiology in autism. *Pathophysiology.* 1997; 4:1485-8.

Date	Events at the Royal Free	Events at the UK Department of Health	Events at The Lancet	Relevant scientific publications other than from Royal Free	Events in the national media	Events at the GMC
February - July 1997	Paper written and submitted to *The Lancet* by July (confirmed by documents in evidence at GMC including statement of *Lancet* deputy editor Dr. John Bignall to GMC).[20]					
March 19, 1997			*Lancet* contact Barr of Dawbarns legal firm with complaint over copyright.			
March 1997			Barr writes to Horton highlighting reference to AW's role in MMR litigation.			
March 19, 1997	AW corresponds with dean over LAB funding research. Grant remains in suspense account.					
March 26, 1997	BMA ethics committee dismiss dean's concerns over LAB pilot study.					

[20] GMC vs Wakefield, Walker-Smith and Murch. Statement of Dr. John Bignall to GMC. September 13, 2005. Page 1, paras 2-4.

Date			BBC Newsnight
			Barr reports " getting help from the team at the Royal Free and experts all over the world who were looking into what was happening."
May 2, 1997	JCVI receives reports of children having **developmental and communication problems**, specifically **after MMR.** JCVI's determination: "These reports represent parental perception of vaccine associated problems; health professionals were likely to show a more consistent pattern of reporting." That is, concerns dismissed. This is almost 1 year before *The Lancet* paper is published.		
July 1997			
September 1997	Meeting at AW's request with Tessa Jowell, Minister of Health, with lawyers and parent representatives. AW asks Minister for meeting of independent experts to review the MMR data.	Proposed meeting taken over by Chief Medical Officer, Sir Kenneth Calman, who rejects the independent scientists recommended by AW.	

Date	Events at the Royal Free	Events at the UK Department of Health	Events at The Lancet	Relevant scientific publications other than from Royal Free	Events in the national media	Events at the GMC
September 4, 1997	LAB funding transferred from suspense account in medical school to Special Trustees charitable account in the Royal Free Hospital by the dean.					
October 1997	LAB-funded viral detection study starts.					
January 12, 1998	AW writes to colleagues about position on MMR and single (monovalent) vaccines.					
January 22, 1998	Dean responds to AW urging support for **monovalent** vaccines.					
February 28, 1998	The dean's press briefing is held. AW recommends **monovalent** vaccines.		"That Paper" published in *The Lancet*.		International media attention.	
March 4, 1998			Rouse letter sent to *The Lancet* referring to "litigation bias."	Weibel et al. describe permanent brain damage following MMR vaccination in the US National Vaccine Injury Compensation Program.[21]		

[21] Weibel RE, Caserta V, Benor DE. Acute encephalopathy followed by permanent brain injury or death associated with further attenuated measles vaccines: A review of claims submitted to the National Vaccine Injury Compensation Program, *Paediatrics.* 1998;101:383-387.

Date			
April 26, 1998	"George" the Whistleblower meets Barr and assistant Limb on Newcastle station		
May 2, 1998		Altered Rouse letter plus AW's response appear in *The Lancet*	
August 1998	Department of Health withdraws licenses for single vaccines despite unprecedented demand.[22]		
February 28, 1999	Second meeting with "George" on Newcastle station with Barr, Limb, and AW. George reiterates previous claims.		
September 1999	LAB pilot study completed.		
January 2000			Plesner from Denmark publishes follow up study of MMR complications. Confirms that severe ataxias are associated with "**residual cognitive deficits in some children.**"[23]
2000–2005	Further papers published on bowel disease in autism from the Royal Free.		

22 Buncombe A. (1998, September 1). Measles jab withdrawn due to 'high demand'. The Independent. Retrieved from http://www.independent.co.uk/news/measles-jab-withdrawn-due-to-high-demand-1195247.html

23 Plesner AM, Hansen FJ, Taadon K, Nielson LH, Larsen CB, Pedersen E. Gait disturbance interpreted as cerebellar ataxia after MMR vaccination at 15 months of age: a follow-up study. *Acta Paediatrica.* 2000;89:58–63.

Date	Events at the Royal Free	Events at the UK Department of Health	Events at The Lancet	Relevant scientific publications other than from Royal Free	Events in the national media	Events at the GMC
October 31, 2001	AW leaves RFH.					
February 11, 2002	AW writes to Chief Medical Officer urging a further meeting to discuss vaccine safety concerns. Request declined.					
February 18, 2004			Deer meets with Horton. (a.m.) Senior authors of The Lancet paper meet with Horton. (p.m.)		AW meets with editorial staff of The Sunday Times.	
February 20, 2004					Horton declares Lancet paper "fatally flawed."	
February 22, 2004						Allegations published by The Sunday Times.[24]
February 25, 2004						Deer files complaint to UK's General Medical Council (GMC).
March 6, 2004			Retraction of an interpretation" published in The Lancet.[25]			

[24] Revealed: MMR Research Scandal Brian Deer. (2004, February 22). The Sunday Times.
[25] Murch, et al. Retraction of an interpretation. The Lancet. 2004 Mar 6;363(9411):750.

September 2004			
2006	Horton publishes *MMR: Science and Fiction* where he admits assisting GMC in prosecution of AW and colleagues.		GMC appoints Professor McDevitt as chairman of Fitness to Practice panel. McDevitt sat on the JCVI during the time the dangerous MMR was used. McDevitt failed to declare this conflict of interest. He was removed from the panel.
July 16, 2007			GMC proceedings start.
February 8, 2009			Deer publishes further false claims in *Sunday Times* "MMR doctor Andrew Wakefield fixed data on autism."[26]
January 28, 2010			GMC issues findings on facts.
February 2, 2010		Full retraction of 1998 paper published by *The Lancet*.	

[26] Deer B. (2009, February 8) MMR doctor Andrew Wakefield fixed data on autism. *The Sunday Times*.

Postscript

by James Moody, Esq.

We read in Sir Graham Wilson's classic book *The Hazards of Immunization:*[1] "It is for us and for those who come after us to see that the sword which vaccines and antisera have put into our hands is never allowed to tarnish through overconfidence, negligence, carelessness, or want of foresight." In *Callous Disregard*, Dr. Andy Wakefield has revealed the details of his ongoing mission to heed this warning.

Although improvements in sanitation, nutrition, and clinical care in our advanced post-industrial civilization had reduced much of the burden of infectious disease, vaccines continued to be promoted as the "weapon" of choice in the war against disease.

As with any war, there are casualties (beginning with the truth), and this is also the case in the war against infection. A small number of casualties are inevitable — and some argue this is justifiable due to the purported overall benefits to society. But we have a moral, ethical, and legal duty to minimize the collateral damage and to take good care of the innocent victims (including providing compensation) in this war against infection. The "communitarian" wing of public health has decided that the good of the many supplants the ethical obligations owed to each child. Some public health officials have accepted an unknown burden of chronic disease — especially autism but also other immune, autoimmune, and developmental disorders — as a fair trade for the prevention of acute morbidity and mortality from infection. Epidemic rates of autism,[2] compelling anecdotal evidence of lower autism rates in unvaccinated populations (e.g., non-vaccinating Amish families[3]) and a lack of baseline data comparing the health histories of vaccinated versus unvaccinated children, together signal an urgent need to reassess the acceptability of a "greater good" vaccine policy. A crucial gap in our vaccine safety science was recently recognized by the US National Vaccine Advisory Committee.[4] And the Centers for Disease Control (CDC) guards its Vaccine Safety Datalink database statistics seemingly as tightly as our military leaders guard our country's nuclear secrets.

Without transparency and data, it is simply impossible to conclude how much chronic illness, including autism, is caused by vaccines.

The terrible tragedy of epic proportion is that most of the autism epidemic (and other chronic adverse reactions) could have been prevented by changes in the vaccine schedule, formulation and screening, as well as an ongoing program of comparative baseline research in humans and primates. I speculate that the motive for the cover-up and the ongoing government policy of "deliberate ignorance" is most likely the fear that honesty about chronic vaccine adverse events would increasingly tempt parents to forego the risks and rely upon the purported herd immunity of others. (Herd immunity itself is in question because there have been disease outbreaks even in highly vaccinated populations.) Without honest investigation, transparency and disclosure, can there truly be informed consent?

As you have read in this book, the US vaccine court began compensating and the US Department of Health and Human Services began secretly settling cases of vaccine caused autism since 1991, including the quiet concession of liability in the case of Hannah Poling,[5] one of the "test" cases in the Omnibus Autism Proceeding. There also was a settlement for MMR-caused autism in the 2002 Hiatt case ($5.1 million)[6] and most recently the Bailey Banks case.[7] The precedent for the admission of vaccine-induced autism is there; what remains to be resolved is the body count, appropriate treatments, and reform of the vaccine schedule to prevent autism and other vaccine caused chronic disorders.

With a history including the clandestine meeting between US regulators and industry at the Simpsonwood Retreat Center in Norcross, GA, in 2000;[8] highly biased and ineffectual Institute of Medicine "reviews" of vaccine safety in 2001 and 2004; and a deeply flawed string of "studies" reminiscent of the junk epidemiology once used to defend tobacco safety, all as water under the bridge, the CDC eventually admitted that its epidemiology was flawed[9] and, in a leaked media strategy document, that it did not have the science to dispel safety questions of "anti-vaccine" challengers.[10]

Dr. Wakefield has been attacked in an orchestrated campaign to "discredit" him and his research, an attack which included the longest running "show trial" in the history of the UK's licensing body, the General Medical Council (GMC). Sadly, this "kangaroo court" was an orgy of prosecutorial misconduct, false testimony, and mischaracterization of appropriate clinical care of desperately sick children spun as "unethical" research. In one of the more bizarre incidents of this skirmish, the announcement of the retraction of *The Lancet* paper following the January 28, 2010, GMC findings was proclaimed at the February 4, 2010, meeting of the National Vaccine Advisory Committee (which advises the Secretary of Health and Human Services on vaccine policy). This was greeted with cheers and "high fives" from the federal and public health elite in attendance. My public comment at the end of the meeting simply pointed out that this Orwellian effort to erase history and the contributions made to science by these 12 children will not succeed.

Dr. Wakefield is the "Ralph Nader of vaccine safety." He is the latest in a long line of scientists who use the power of the scientific method to challenge establishment orthodoxy. Thanks to Galileo, Semmelweiss, Needleman, and McBride, we now take it for granted that the Earth is not the center of the Universe, that doctors must wash their hands to prevent the spread of infection, that lead impairs neurological development in children, and that thalidomide causes birth defects. And now, thanks to Dr. Wakefield, we will one day have safer vaccines and better treatments for autism.

Endnotes

[1] Wilson G. *The Hazards of Immunization*. London: The Athlone Press, 1967.

[2] http://www.cdc.gov/ncbddd/autism/addm.html.

[3] Blaxill M. (2008, May 14). Olmsted, the Amish and Autism. Part One. Retrieved from http://www.ageofautism.com/2008/05/olsted-the-amis.html.

Blaxill M. (2008, May 15). Olmsted, the Amish and Autism. Part Two. Retrieved from

http://www.ageofautism.com/2008/05/olsted-the-am-1.html

[4] NVAC. (2009, June 2). "Recommendations on the Centers for Disease Control and Prevention Immunization Safety Office Draft 5-Year Scientific Agenda. (see in particular recommendation #7). Retrieved from http://www.hhs.gov/nvpo/nvac/ NVACRecommendationsISOScientificAgendaFinal.pdf.

[5] Kirby D. (2008, February 26). The Vaccine Court Document Every American Should Read. *Huffington Post*. Retrieved from http://www.huffingtonpost.com/david kirby/the vaccineautism court _b_88558.html.

CBS News. Retrieved from http://www.cbsnews.com/sections/primarysource/ main501263.shtml?contributor=41919.

[6] Taylor G. (2008, March 9). Phil and Misty Hiatt: We Were Compensated Too. Adventures in Autism. Retrieved from http://adventuresinautism.blogspot. com/2008/03/phil and misty hiatt we were.html.

[7] Kennedy R, Kirby D. (2009, February 24). Vaccine Court: Autism Debate Continues. *Huffington Post*. Retrieved from http://www.huffingtonpost.com/robert f kennedy jr and david kirby/vaccine court autism deba_b_169673.html.

[8] See http://www.safeminds.org/government-affairs/foia/simpsonwood.html.

[9] Kirby D. (2008, June 21). CDC: Vaccine Study Used Flawed Methods. *Huffington Post*. Retrieved from http://www.huffingtonpost.com/david kirby/cdc vaccine study used fl_b_108462.html.

[10] Moody J. (2009, August 5). CDC Media Plan Shocker — We Don't Have the Science — Some claims against vaccine cannot be disproved. *Age of Autism*. Retrieved from http://www.ageofautism.com/2009/08/cdc media plan shocker we don't have the science some claims against vaccine cannot be disproved .html.

BIOGRAPHY

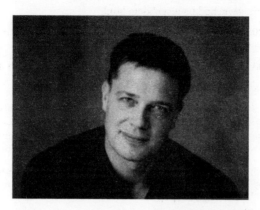

Photo credit: Vibeke Dahl

Andrew Wakefield, MB, BS, FRCS, FRCPath, is an academic gastroenterologist. He received his medical degree from St. Mary's Hospital Medical School (part of the University of London) in 1981, one of the third generation of his family to have studied medicine at that teaching hospital. He pursued a career in gastrointestinal surgery with a particular interest in inflammatory bowel disease. He qualified as Fellow of the Royal College of Surgeons in 1985 and in 1996 was awarded a Wellcome Trust Traveling Fellowship to study small intestinal transplantation in Toronto, Canada. He was made a Fellow of the Royal College of Pathologists in 2001. He has published over 130 original scientific articles, book chapters, and invited scientific commentaries.

In the pursuit of possible links between childhood vaccines, intestinal inflammation, and neurologic injury in children, Dr. Wakefield lost his job in the Department of Medicine at London's Royal Free Hospital, his country, his career, and his medical license.

He is married to Carmel, a physician and a classical radio presenter. He has four children, James, Sam, Imogen, and Corin, and a black mongrel called Bella.